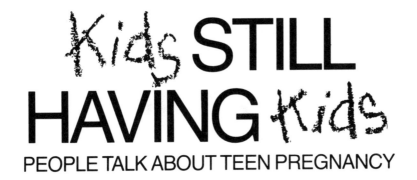

Kids STILL HAVING Kids

PEOPLE TALK ABOUT TEEN PREGNANCY

BY JANET BODE

ART BY STAN MACK

FRANKLIN WATTS
NEW YORK/CHICAGO/LONDON/TORONTO/SYDNEY

TO SCOTT

Library of Congress Cataloging-in-Publication Data
Bode, Janet.
Kids still having kids: people talk about teen pregnancy/by Janet Bode
p. cm.
Includes bibliographical references and index.
Summary: Presents interviews with teenage mothers and provides
information about adoption, parenting, abortion, and foster care.
ISBN 0-531-11132-6. — ISBN 0-531-15254-5 (trade)
1. Teenagers—United States—Sexual behavior—Juvenile literature.
2. Teenage pregnancy—United States—Juvenile literature.
3. Teenage parents—United States—Juvenile literature.
[1. Pregnancy. 2. Teenage parents. 3. Sex instruction for youth.]
I. Title.
HQ27.B618 1992
306.85'6–dc20   92-14175 CIP AC

ACKNOWLEDGMENTS

Many thanks to my family for their continual support: Stan Mack, Carl Bode, Barbara Bode, Carolyn Bode, Frieda Lutze, Ernie Lutze. And thanks, too, to my friends: Wendy Caplan, Chas Carner, Lucy Cefalu, Jeanne Dougherty, Andrea Eagan, Kay Franey, Ted Gottfried, Carole Mayedo, Marvin Mazor, Rosemarie Mazor, Judy Pollock, Mike Sexton, Kate Sullivan.

I also received invaluable assistance from these sources: Andrea Rose Askowitz and Veena Cabreros-Sud, SOS, New York City; Maria Delgado, Marie Jean, and Yoli Rojas, New York City Department of Health, Bureau of School Children and Adolescent Health, City Volunteer Corps; Martha Kuss, Media Specialist, Crawford High School, San Diego, California; Amy Miller, M.D., Director, Chemically Abusing Problem Adolescence Program, Trinity House of St. Luke's-Roosevelt Hospital, New York City; Lynn Paltrow, American Civil Liberties Union/Reproductive Freedom Project, New York City; Tamar Raphael, Feminist Majority, Arlington, Virginia; Ellen Ramsay, Media Specialist, Amphitheater High School, Tucson, Arizona; Susan Tew, The Alan Guttmacher Institute, New York City; Cynthia Wilson, Office of Adolescent Parenting Program, LYFE, New York City.

And thank you to the teenagers who shared their stories. This book wouldn't have been possible without you.

Also by Janet Bode

BEATING THE ODDS: Stories of Unexpected Achievers
DIFFERENT WORLDS:
Interracial and Cross-Cultural Dating
NEW KIDS ON THE BLOCK:
Oral Histories of Immigrant Teens
TRUCE: Ending the Sibling War
THE VOICES OF RAPE

CONTENTS

PART I

Sex

"DON'T READ THIS BOOK!"

"A parent wants [Howard] county middle school libraries to remove the book, *Kids Having Kids: The Unwed Teenage Parent*, by Janet Bode, which uses case histories to discuss decisions made by pregnant teenagers, including adoption and abortion."

"'It is not fit for a young girl or boy to be reading this book,' the parent said."

THE BALTIMORE SUN,
October 23, 1990.[1]

When I wrote *Kids Having Kids*, my goal was simple. I wanted to give information to teenagers who were pregnant by mistake. That way, I thought, they'd be a step closer to being able to decide what to do next.

I was proud of the book. Teenagers from across the country sent me letters saying that reading about other teens who dealt with this problem helped them solve their own. The book won awards.

I never thought that people would try to ban it. But they did. My first reaction was, why would anyone want to keep teenagers ignorant of the facts?

I've learned a lot since then.

Particularly when it comes to children and teenagers, some people say there should not be a free flow of information. We must protect kids. Others call that censorship.

When the publisher asked me if I'd write a new book on the topic of pregnancy among teenagers, I thought it was a good idea. This time, though, I wondered—should I change how I decide what to include and what to leave out?

Before I write on any subject, I talk to people, both in groups and one-on-one. I tape-record facts and opinions, advice and decisions. I interview not only teenagers, but also adults involved in the issue.

For this book, *Kids Still Having Kids*, I heard from teens who are made pregnant by a stepfather, an uncle, a brother. Do I cut that information? Some people don't want to know that incest exists. And they especially don't want teenagers to read about it.

What about accounts from those who become pregnant at eleven? Are parents that age too young to mention? Will some readers get upset? Will they think I'm saying it's okay to have sex at any age?

And, of course, if there is a section on abortion, will some people automatically demand that this book be kept from teenagers' hands? By far, the most complaints to my publisher and to librarians came because I included abortion as an option for a girl with an unwanted pregnancy.

I make choices—the way I always have.

I have opinions. I'm human. I try, though, to present a balanced picture. I look for patterns and trends. I go after the most current and accurate information.

No single teenager's interview is included unless she or he mirrors the accounts I heard from others. No adult's words are reported unless I saw that they, too, represent the views of many others.

The world is not perfect. I wish there weren't any accounts of unwanted pregnancies and child abuse and failed foster care and other such tragedies. But there are, and not writing about them won't make these problems go away. In fact, only by examining them can we hope to find solutions.

I didn't write this book to offend or to outrage. I wrote it to give you, the teenage reader, a place to start when confronting a surprise pregnancy—or even one you planned. Here is information from adult experts and here are real-life examples of how your peers are handling similar situations.

I believe we can learn from others. By hearing what knowledgeable adults have to say, combined with details from teens on how they found solutions, your own path may be made easier.

This is a book more of stories than statistics. Come along with me as I ask different individuals about love, sex, and, especially, what they did if or when pregnancy touched their lives.

What was your life like before the pregnancy, I begin. What happened after that? How did you make decisions about what to do? How did you tell your family and friends? What was the reaction? What have you learned from this experience? What advice do you have for others?

The voices you hear are the voices I heard. The grammar isn't always perfect, but I think the meaning is always clear.

To protect the identity of the teenagers who speak on these pages, I have changed their names and a few other details. I guarantee them this privacy in exchange for their letting you and me in their lives. The adults are named and their job titles given.

This is a book that you don't have to read from beginning to end. Look at the contents pages and see if any of the chapters speak to you.

Let's say you're pregnant and considering adoption. Start with the sections on adoption, parenting, and foster care. If your girlfriend has just told you she's pregnant, first turn to the parts that are aimed at fathers-to-be and fathers.

If you haven't had sex, or if you're writing a paper,

begin with the boxed information. Inside those rectangles are facts and figures about teen pregnancy and related issues, for nonparents and parents alike.

Surprise pregnancies can happen to anyone, even you. If this is the case, keep the following in mind.

You are not alone. People will help you. Start today to gather information and to ask for advice from those you respect. You want to make wise decisions about what to do.

And finally, *not* making a decision is making a decision. For yourself and your future—get started.

"my girlfriend says, 'a virgin wouldn't understand.'"

AMBER, 16 YEARS OLD

My best girlfriend makes me crazy. She's smart except about guys. Every other month she comes to me and says she thinks she's pregnant. I say, "Didn't you learn anything last time?"

She says, "I didn't think. We were so caught up in it...."

She tells me she'd feel weird discussing birth control with her boyfriend. I say, "You're close enough to have sex. You're not close enough to talk with him about birth control?"

"You're a virgin," she says. "You wouldn't understand. It just doesn't feel the same if you use a rubber."

"Maybe you trust your boyfriend. But you're the one who's going to get pregnant."

"Nothing's going to happen to me," she always answers.

"Everyone's having sex but me."

LORENZO, 18 YEARS OLD

There's a lot of pressure to have sex. And there's a lot of curiosity. It's hard to have self-control. So some teenagers *rush*. They don't think that sex is more than sex.

To me, it's a bonding between two people. It's very intimate. It's about making a commitment.

I'm eighteen and I haven't had sex. I'm sure guys hit sixteen, seventeen, eighteen, and they say, "Oh, I stopped being a virgin when I was fifteen."

They exaggerate so they won't feel out of place. They think, "Everyone's having sex but me." Sometimes I feel that way.

I have a group of friends and they're all having sex. Fathers tell sons, "Have sex, and enjoy yourself." They think it's the manly thing to do.

A couple of months ago, my friends, like, found someone for me to have sex with. They were all set to go. I knew I had an expression on my face. They could guess it would be my first time. They started laughing and saying, "You're a virgin." I didn't know whether to hide it or fake it.

I thought of my mother. She says if a guy has sex with a girl and she gets pregnant, she goes through a lot. And I would, too. How can I take the chance of having a child when I'm not even settled myself?

WHO'S HAVING SEX[2]

AGE	FEMALES	MALES
15	27%	33%
16	34%	50%
17	52%	66%
18	70%	72%
19	78%	86%

[No national surveys include percentage having sex for those 11 through 14 years old.]

Half of all teen females are pregnant because of coercion. That means force and pressure.

I ask the ones I see in my practice, "Did you initiate the sex?"

The answer: "Not really."

"Did you try to stop it?"

"Yes, but not enough."

"Was it rape?"

"Well, no. It's just easier to do it than to say 'no' and have to fight."

The details start. They've been going out for a while. Her parents are away. She and the boyfriend are getting into it. His hand is on her breast. Her hand is down his pants.

She wants to do it. But she's not sure. She's getting nervous. She wonders, Can I change my mind?

"Of course," I tell her.

"When do you know when to stop?" she asks.

That's the question you have to think about *before* you have sex.

People say, "Well, if teenagers have sex, why don't they use birth control? It's so easy." What they forget is that it's a whole scenario.

Even if it's only a male going to the store to buy con-

BIRTH CONTROL ODDS[3]

Sex with birth control is safer than sex without birth control. But how effective are the different methods?
In the first year of sexual activity, 85% of females using no birth control become pregnant.
Using condoms: 10% to 18% become pregnant
Diaphragms or cervical caps: 12% to 39%
Sponge containing spermicide: 16% to 52%
Pill: 4% to 9%
IUDs (intrauterine devices): 2.5% to 4.5%
Shots (injectable contraceptives): 0.4%
Implants (Norplant): 0.05% to 0.5%

doms, he has to put up with comments like, "I'll have to charge you an entertainment tax."

A female goes in and she hears, "Hey, honey, you're not the one who's supposed to be buying these." She gets embarrassed.

For the female to get on the pill, get a diaphragm, a cervical cap, whatever her choice, she has to become part of the medical system. She has to find time for a doctor's appointment, show up, probably wait, undress, get up on a table, put her legs in stirrups....

This is what "getting birth control" means. Lots of teens think it's too much of a hassle. Of course, getting pregnant is an even bigger hassle.

"If you really love me...!"

SARAH, 17 YEARS OLD

I sleep with my boyfriend, and to me it's a *big deal*. But he just tried to get me pregnant. *I couldn't believe it*! I figured he was going to use the withdrawal method. He didn't. I said, "How could you maybe ruin my life without asking me first?"

He kept saying, "I want there to be something between us. If you really love me, you'll give me a baby."

"I'm not a baby machine," I told him.

At the same time, though, he's changed. He never stands me up anymore. He buys me things. It feels good to have someone who's ALWAYS there and thinks I'm great. It gives me confidence. I can't help loving him.

My period is irregular, so I'm not *that* worried it's late.

SEXUALLY TRANSMITTED DISEASES (STDS)[4]

CHLAMYDIA: Young women 15 to 19 may have the highest infection rate of any age group. It can cause sterility among men, as well as women.

GENITAL WARTS: As many as a third of all sexually active teenagers may be infected. They can lead to cervical cancer.

HERPES: The infection rate may be increasing. Herpes has no cure and can cause miscarriage, stillbirth, and damage to infants during childbirth.

SYPHILIS: The infection rate for those age 15 to 19 has jumped 67 percent since 1985. If untreated, the person may develop heart disease, blindness, and mental incapacity. Syphilis can cause damage to infants during childbirth.

AIDS: One percent of all reported AIDS cases involve teenagers, but a fifth of all people with AIDS are in their twenties. There is no cure.

SEX, DRUGS, AIDS, AND PREGNANCY

AIDS is caused by the human immunodeficiency virus (HIV). In most cases, the virus is transmitted when you have unprotected sex with someone who is infected or when you share nonsterile needles to shoot drugs.

Since the epidemic started, 670 teenagers aged 13 to 19 have developed AIDS, as have 7,097 people aged 20 to 24. It is estimated that for every known case of AIDS, there are ten more people infected with HIV. That means about 78,000 people between 13 and 24 may now be HIV-positive. The average time between becoming infected and developing AIDS is five to ten years. In other words, a 21-year-old with AIDS was probably exposed to the virus sometime between the ages of 11 and 16.

While more than half the AIDS cases among 13- to 24-year-olds involve gay or bisexual males, the number of heterosexual teen females is slowly increasing.[5] Those most likely to be infected shoot drugs or have sex with males who do or with bisexuals.

For complete protection against HIV and AIDS, don't have sex and don't share hypodermic needles. If you have sex, start by making safe sex as natural and automatic as fastening your seat belt when you get into a car. Use condoms every time the penis enters the vagina, anus, or mouth. You want to prevent the virus from getting into your body.

If you shoot drugs, either don't share the needle and works or clean them first. (Soak them in a mixture of water and bleach or water and alcohol for fifteen minutes. Rinse them in water afterwards. You don't want to shoot bleach or alcohol into your blood.)

If you become pregnant and are infected with HIV or have AIDS, you have tough choices to make. Consider these questions: Will continuing the pregnancy make me sicker or shorten my life? Have I been taking any medication that could damage the fetus? If I get sick or if I die, who will care for the baby? If the baby gets sick or dies, can I cope? Studies show that 13 to 30 percent of babies born to HIV-positive mothers end up with the virus, too.[6]

For more information about AIDS and pregnancy, call 1-800-342-AIDS (English); 1-800-344-SIDA (Spanish).

JAN STOLLENWERK, SCHOOL NURSE,
SAN DIEGO, CALIFORNIA

A student came to my office, sat down, and said, "I think I'm pregnant."

"Oh, really?" I said, as we checked the calendar to see when she had her last period. "Do you have sex often?"

"No, this was my first time."

"When? "

"Saturday night."

This was Monday morning. I said, "Well, according to your menstrual cycle, I don't think you're pregnant right now. But you know what? That egg is just sitting there ready to pop out of the ovary. And that sperm is just sitting in the fallopian tube waiting for it.

"You might not be pregnant now, but it can happen any minute."

"Any minute? Oh, my gosh."

"Did you use protection—birth control?"

"Yes," she said, "but it fell off."

That means they didn't use anything.

"Does your boyfriend love you?" I said.

"Oh, yes."

"If you were out in the parking lot together and some guy came up and hit you, would he protect you?"

"*Oh, yes.* He'd punch his lights out."

"Why?"

"Why? He doesn't want me to get hurt."

I said, "Tell me. Did your boyfriend have a good time Saturday night?"

"Yes."

"Did you have a good time?"

"It was okay."

"Is your boyfriend out in the lunch court now?"

"Yes."

"Is he having a good time?"

"I guess so."

"Are you having a good time right now?"

"No."

"Are you going to have a good time tomorrow? What about for the next two weeks until your period comes? Are you going to have a good time?"

"No. I'm going to be worried about whether I'm pregnant."

"So you're worrying and hurting. Isn't it hurting you?"

"Yes."

I said, "Isn't this the same thing? Why doesn't your boyfriend take precaution and protection to keep you from all this pain you're going through right now? If he would protect you from a stranger hitting you, wouldn't he also want to protect you from this fear of pregnancy?"

"Well, yes, he would."

"Exactly. You want to be protected. He should be the protector."

	ARE YOU USING BIRTH CONTROL?[7]
○	In a study, only two or three in ten sexually active teenagers regularly used birth control. When the rest were asked why they weren't using any protection, nearly one in ten said they were trying to get pregnant or were already pregnant. Four in ten thought they couldn't become pregnant because it was the "wrong time of the month." The others didn't expect to have sex, were afraid to have a pelvic exam, or thought they were too young to become pregnant.

PART II

Pregnant

" Pregnant ? I'm only eleven. "

YVELINE, 21 YEARS OLD

"I remember the day that I got my first period. It was right before I turned ten.

I started bleeding when I woke up. Me and my sister used to sleep in the same bed. So she was the only one who knew. I was scared to tell my mother. I didn't know if she would kill me.

My sister kept saying, "We've gotta tell. We've gotta tell."

"No," I said. But she did anyway.

I went in the bathroom. My mother was there. She had pads in her hands and told me to go clean up.

"You're a woman now," she said. "You have to be very careful."

My mother is old-fashioned. You're not supposed to question your parents about anything. Especially sex. You'll get smacked if you do. The thought is, if it's meant for you to know, they'll tell you.

I never brought up the issue of my period or sex again and neither did she. After that bleeding, though, I became *totally* curious. There's more to this than I knew.

I had girlfriends at school, but no one that I spoke to about my feelings. I couldn't ask them.

I would have felt comfortable asking my father. But he lived in Haiti. I lived in Brooklyn. Since my parents divorced, I communicated with him through letters. I'd write him and give the letters to my mother to mail. I never knew whether she was reading what I said.

I missed my father. And my mother was never home. She worked long hours to support us.

When I was younger and lived with my father, he used to *always* be there. When I was eleven and a half and had sex for the first time, I felt like I was communicating with my father again. Now, don't get confused. I never had sex with my dad. It was just, to me, having sex meant being close to a male.

Having sex also was painful and scary. I didn't know what I was doing. Nor did the guy. We just did it.

The second time, I got pregnant. That's the only detail I remember. And don't ask me questions about the guy. He was no one important in my life.

At first, I didn't know I was pregnant. I kept having my period. Normally I would have it for five days. That May, the year my sister got her first communion, I only bled for two days.

I thought, "As long as I'm bleeding, I'm fine."

Anyway, my stepmother had once told me, "Babies are dropped from the sky and fall into your stomach. After you get married, you're ready to have a baby. God decides when."

I couldn't get pregnant. I wasn't married.

I went home to Haiti that summer and stayed for about a month and a half. "Is everything okay?" my stepmother said. My hips were growing. My breasts were growing. Anyone else would think, it's puberty. Forming out, like you're supposed to.

"You just don't *look* right," my stepmother said.

"I'm okay," I told her. From then on, I kept her quiet by asking for pads.

By the time I got back to Brooklyn, I started feeling self-conscious. Before that, when my sister and I showered, my mother prepared our clothes and we went to her room to get dressed. We walked around each other naked. It was no big deal.

Now I was covering myself. I felt *huge*.

"You never did that before," my mother said.

"My stepmother told me, 'You have stepbrothers around here. Cover yourself. You're a lady.'"

"You don't have stepbrothers here," my mother said, and she pulled off the towel. *"What's that?!"*

I had a line from my belly button to my breasts.

"Put on your clothes. You're going to the doctor!"

I'll never forget the hospital. There were five doctors in the room with me. They kept poking at my body. It hurt.

One doctor said, "I'm sure it didn't hurt when you opened your legs."

Another doctor, an Oriental lady, told me to get dressed. She took me in her office and started showing me books about people giving birth. "Do you know about this?" she asked me.

I didn't.

She told me what abortion was. What adoption was. What having a baby was like.

After I left her office, she asked my mother to go in. They were in there for maybe five minutes. When my mother came out, I could see smoke pouring out of her ears. She slapped me and said, "We're going home."

"You need to return tomorrow," the doctor said as we walked to the elevator.

We went back for the results of the urine and blood tests. I was almost five months pregnant. "What do you want to do?" the doctor asked my mother.

"I want her to have an abortion."

"We can't do it. It would be risky. Your daughter's too young and too many weeks pregnant. She waited too long."

"*I don't care!*" my mother screamed. "Nothing's going to happen to her. She'll be fine."

The doctor refused.

See, my mother was ill at that time. She was going to the hospital a lot. I think it was even causing some mental problems. At that time, she lost her job, lost the house to the bank, lost everything.

The next thing I knew a social worker came to the house. They took me and my sister to family court. The judge asked, did I want to go home? "No," I said, "I'm scared of my mother." She was *very* upset with me. I thought she might beat me.

The court sent me to Louise Wise, a shelter for unwed mothers. Of the twelve of us there, I was the youngest. The other girls called me cry baby. I was depressed about everything.

I didn't like the changes in my body. I felt heavy, fat, like I couldn't move. We had mandatory exercise classes. Lamaze method childbirth classes. Breathing classes. I was told if I didn't do them, giving birth would be painful. Sometimes, though, I wasn't in the mood.

We had chores to do, too. We took turns cooking. The food was delicious. After that first month, things got better. One of the workers would stick up for me. I could come to her office and talk whenever I wanted.

There was a regular school just for us. We'd go every day. I wanted to keep up in those classes. I always had ambition. I had started seventh grade.

I was strongly thinking about adoption. The social workers were pushing it. They didn't come out and say, "I think you should give up your child." But I could tell that's what they thought.

I was getting scared of childbirth. I heard women talk about Eve and how this was punishment from God. "Labor is the most painful thing that can happen to a woman," they'd say.

I never heard anyone say raising a child is more difficult than having a baby. I would soon find out....
(To be continued in Part VI: Parents)

BONNIE GROH, TEEN-PARENT DIRECTOR,

DELTA SCHOOLCRAFT INTERMEDIATE

SCHOOL DISTRICT, ESCANABA, MICHIGAN

Nine percent of teen mothers attempt suicide. That's about seven times the national rate for teenage girls who are not mothers. I worry about that.

There are many reasons that teens get pregnant. If yours is a surprise pregnancy, you need to think about why it happened. You don't want to become pregnant again for the same reason.

Maybe you decided to get pregnant as a way out of the house. Or you live romantically. You thought if you have *his* baby, you are showing your love. He will be yours forever.

Or maybe you felt this is how you can become successful. You've been cut down before. You don't feel cared for. If you have a baby, you'll be accepted. And you can turn around and really care for someone else, that child.

Most likely, you don't want to become pregnant. Let's say you even take the pill, one of the safest and most popular birth control methods. But maybe you weren't careful to take it every day about the same time.

Or you had the flu and threw up in the morning. You didn't know that meant the pill wasn't absorbed like it should be. Then if you had sex, you should use two methods of protection.

○	**SEE A DOCTOR**[2] More than half the expectant teens don't get any prenatal care during their first trimester. One in ten doesn't get care until her third trimester. Early and thorough medical attention can prevent low birth weight, a major factor contributing to infant death.

Now your period hasn't come. Your breasts are sore. You're pregnant.

You *still* have choices.

You can go on with the pregnancy and keep the child.

You can relinquish the child for adoption.

You can turn to foster care and place the child in a temporary home until you're more ready for parenting.

You can have an abortion and end the pregnancy.

I work at an educational institution that gets federal funds, so we can't talk either for or against abortion. But when I have teenage girls in conflict, I ask them, "What do you think are your choices?" Usually they bring up these options, including abortion.

There's one other choice they mention, too: do or don't I want to get married? Today most of you are choosing not to get married.

If you're pregnant, you should see someone you feel good talking to—a favorite teacher, a counselor, a doctor, a parent you can count on to give you correct advice.

You might feel you can't have family involvement until you decide what you want to do. In that case, talk to some adult you trust. Whether a pregnancy is planned or unplanned, making decisions about what to do is a lot to handle, especially on your own.

The decisions you make should be part of a plan. Impulse decisions simply force you to deal with the consequences later. Start planning what to do about a pregnancy by answering these questions:

- How do I feel about the direction I'm going in life?
- What are my goals?
- Are those goals possible if I have a child now?
- Is medical care easy to get and affordable where I live?
- Can I stick with my schooling if I have a child?
- If my eating habits aren't the best, am I willing to change them and eat well during and after the pregnancy?
- Is the father around? Is he supportive? Will he be supportive five or ten years from now?
- Do the two of us share the same values and feelings about the importance of the family, and how to take care of and raise a child?
- Can one or both of us get a decent job so we won't have to live in poverty?
- Am I compulsive about spending or am I good at stretching the dollar? Can I cover my expenses for food, clothing, and rent—plus for a child?
- Will my family be there as part of my support system?
- Will they still help out once the child is a toddler— more adventuresome and harder to raise?
- Is affordable day care available? Will I have to arrange transportation in order to get there? Do they take infants, as well as toddlers and above?
- Do I like caring for a baby? A toddler? A teenager?
- How do I handle my anger and frustration? Would I ever take out my emotions on a child?
- Am I willing to give up lots of my freedom and my social life to take on the responsibility of raising a child— for at least the next eighteen years?
- Can I give a child the future I'd want for him or her?

Making decisions about a surprise pregnancy is painful. It's painful to raise a child. It's painful to relinquish a child for adoption. It's painful to have an abortion. But this doesn't mean you should put off these decisions. Hoping you aren't pregnant won't make it go away.

34

" my birth control failed."

MARISOL, 17 YEARS OLD

I'm the oldest. My mom had me when she was seventeen. I didn't know my real dad until I was ten. Partly, I was raised by my sisters' and brothers' dad. I considered him my father. My real dad is nothing special.

My mom's a single parent now. She works graveyard shift. It's hard financially. She has to get us stuff at the secondhand store. Still, I'm happy with the way she's bringing us up.

One thing I like is she's open about sex. She tells me and my sisters and brothers that it's normal. Every human being gets sexual feelings at certain times with the right person.

And even if it isn't the right person, if we feel we want to experiment—to have intercourse—come to her first. She'd be upset. But that's just being a parent. We should know there are birth-control precautions to take.

I started seeing my boyfriend, Nicholas, three years ago. From the moment we met, I'm thinking, he's *gorgeous*. I'm afraid he thinks I'm just a friend. I put a letter in his car telling him I like him.

He calls me that same day.

My heart starts beating. Fast. I'm embarrassed. "I never thought you'd notice me," I say. He's mellow. He likes country music, caving, hiking where there're trees.

Back then, I'm more like this wild person. Not partying, but I'm up to everything—all the new fads. My hair style is long in back, high and straight up in front. I'm going to school and working forty hours a week at Senn's Boutique. I have money.

He says, "I never expected you to like someone like me. I wanted to ask you out, but I didn't know how."

My friends think we're a really cute couple. They tease, "Oh, let us borrow Nick. He's so sexy."

At first, my mom and him don't hit it off. She doesn't want him to take away her oldest daughter. She gives him the cold shoulder. Next she's trying to like him, but he's Anglo, white. She's Mexican.

My grandmother isn't happy, either. She feels I'm Mexican, I should marry a Mexican guy.

After seeing Nicholas for a while, I know I have these weird feelings—sexual feelings—about him. He's dropping me off at my house after a date. I say to him, "Let's sit on the porch and talk. I have something to ask you."

He keeps looking at my face, going, "What?"

I go, "Nothing. I don't know how to tell you."

"Go ahead."

"I'm embarrassed."

It takes me a half hour to say I have sexual feelings for him. And I don't know if he has the same feelings for me. He say he does, but he doesn't want to pressure me.

"You're not," I say. "I'm the one who brought up the subject. If it's okay, I'll talk to my mom about getting birth control."

The next day I don't plan a speech, I just tell my mom I have to talk to her.

"About what?" she says.

"About me and Nicholas."

I think she has an idea what I'm going to say, but she wants me to come out and say it.

"I'm having sexual feelings for him, and I want to get on birth control."

"Are you sure?" she says.

"Yeah."

"Well, I guess we'll make a doctor's appointment. I want you to know, though, this is hard for me."

Let me tell you, for me, it's hard to go to a GYN for the first time. I think it will be no big deal. Go in. The doctor gives you a prescription for birth control pills. That's it.

Wrong.

My mom keeps telling me, "You're going to have a pap smear."

"What's that?"

She says, "It's a test for cervical cancer. The cervix is at the end of your vagina. You go in the examining room, put your feet up on these stirrup things. The doctor sticks something in you that looks like a duck's beak. He'll stick his fingers in you to check your ovaries and stuff."

"*No way*," I go.

"If you want to be on birth control, yes, he is."

Then she tells me I have to feel my boobs to make sure I don't have lumps, possible breast cancer.

"It's going to be a guy doctor?" I say. And in comes this male doctor. I'm so embarrassed.

My mom stays in the room with me. I want her to. I get through it. I'm sixteen.

The doctor gives me a real pretty case with a butterfly on it that has pills inside. He tells me to take a pill the Sunday after I start my period. Then take it for a month before I have intercourse.

"That's all?" I say.

"Yes, but you might want to use something else as a

precaution not to get pregnant. The pill is about 96 percent to 99 percent effective. Remember, there's always that small percent that fail."

So I'm taking the pills, every day, at the same time. I'm not doing anything wrong. My period is still coming down. But I notice that my pants aren't fitting me any more. My stomach's hurting. I'm nervous.

I go into my mom's room and tell her, "I don't know what's wrong with me." I show her my stomach.

"We'd better make a doctor's appointment."

The doctor tells me to lay down. He looks at my stomach. "You're definitely pregnant."

I go to the laboratory for a blood test. I'm twenty-four weeks pregnant. Not me! I am shocked! I'm that small percent.

Nicholas is excited. *"I'm gonna be a daddy!"* he says, and then he hugs me.

DAVID BERGER, M.D., CHIEF,

DEPARTMENT OF PEDIATRICS,

GOUVERNEUR HOSPITAL, NEW YORK CITY

Teenagers have more problem pregnancies than women in their twenties. More babies born to teen mothers are premature and have low birth weights. Why? An important reason is that once you're pregnant, you don't go to a clinic early and often enough for what's called prenatal care. Prenatal means before the birth.

As soon as you think you might be pregnant, visit a local clinic. You'll learn far more than just that you're expecting. The staff is there to help you give your baby a head start on life. You get common sense counseling, testing, and medical information. Your questions are answered. And in most locations, this prenatal care is free for teenagers.

How often you go to the clinic depends on your needs. If you're healthy and everything is in order, you need to see a health care worker a couple times during the first trimester—the first three months—and three or four times the second trimester. By the third trimester, you have to go more often, usually about every two weeks.

Let's say you're at the clinic. You've learned that a baby can be born with problems based on what you, the mother, are doing to yourself during the pregnancy. You know you shouldn't smoke, drink alcohol, or do illegal drugs. But you might not know that you should also monitor what you eat.

You ask, "Why am I dying for pickles and ice cream in the middle of the night?" We tell you the truth. We have no earthly idea, but it *does* happen. You're normal.

You say, "Since I'm eating for two, is it okay to eat a lot more?" At the most, you should eat five hundred more calories a day. That's a second portion at dinner. You want to gain a total of twenty-five to thirty pounds. And to help you keep track, we weigh you.

You should try to limit an eat-and-run diet of McDonald's. Fast foods have little nutritional value, are often high in fat and salt content, low in iron and other minerals.

Just being low in something like iron is tough on the fetus growing inside you. The baby's blood system is developing, and that takes iron. And you, the mother, may become very iron deficient. By the time you notice any tiredness, weakness, or mental delays remembering things, you and the fetus could be in trouble.

At your prenatal checkups, we give you iron supplements, and you learn what's best to eat. We might tell you, "If you go to McDonald's, stay away from the greasy stuff. Instead order the McLean. Better yet, eat at home and bake or broil your food rather than deep-fat frying it. Eat fruits and vegetables, and if you can't handle certain dairy products, try yogurt or tofu."

During a pregnancy, you go through physical changes. Your pelvic joints loosen, which means the way you walk changes—some call it a duck-walk. If you're brunette, you get a darkening around the face. You may experience swollen legs, feet, and hands, water retention, backaches, and frequent urination, among other things.

At the same time, you go through emotional changes. While each person has somewhat different reactions, as your body changes, your self-image changes. In prenatal care you talk about how you feel about this kind of thing.

You can also discuss how your relationships change with your family, friends, and the father of your child. It's normal for you to have mood swings, to be excited, to be afraid. Every pregnant person goes through that. Even women who want the baby more than anything in the world get nervous and scared and have second thoughts.

At each visit, we look for signs and symptoms of any health problems. For example, we need to know before the delivery if you have diabetes, high blood pressure, or other such conditions. We need to know if you have any sexually transmitted diseases [STDs]—chlamydia, syphilis, gonor-rhea, herpes.

And although we don't routinely test to see if you are HIV-positive or have AIDS, we do what's called a "risk assessment." We tell you your options and let you decide if you want to be tested.

Finally, together, we start planning for the delivery and equally important, what happens after that big day. For yourself, for your child, have regular prenatal visits. It is much more dangerous and complicated if you come in at the last minute when you are due.

"my boyfriend cut out."

COURTNEY, 15 YEARS OLD

In Tucson, where I lived, I liked to hang out at the mall. It was hectic, what with the gangs. There were the Bloods, the Crips, the Alley Raiders, and the Posse.

That's where I first saw Darrell. It was summer. I was fourteen. He was twenty-one.

He was short, dark, and very attractive to me. He was drunk at the time. He had lost his wallet and asked me, did I see it?

I started flirting with him. Then he said, "Take my number and call." So I did.

Almost from the start, we had so much in common it made me crazy. We were both smart and smart asses. We had the same taste in music, old heavy metal.

I found his weak spots. Darrell found mine. Like, I could say something about his age, compared to mine. That would piss him off. He usually dated girls his age or older. I had told him I was seventeen. He almost died when he found out the truth. It hurt his ego.

See, he was a big dope dealer. In fact, that's why he was frantic searching for his wallet. It had $5000 in it. He just forgot he'd tucked it in his pant leg under his sock.

Pretty soon he was coming to stay with me at my house. My bathroom and bedroom, with a queen-size bed, shelves for my clothes, a CD player and TV, were down-stairs. My parents—they adopted me when I was little—lived upstairs. And the downstairs and upstairs were like a completely different house.

My father, a minister—but that's another story—didn't even know Darrell existed. Same for my mother, one busy lady. They would have *shit* if they met him. He had major attitudes towards everybody.

I got pregnant about a month or two after I met him. The day he left town was the day I found out. I stole a pregnancy test and it came out positive. I just knew I'd get pregnant. As many times as we'd been together, of course, I was going to end up that way. I didn't care.

A week later, Darrell called. "You're going to be a father," I said.

He was, like, "Oh, shit."

"So, what are you going to do?"

He said, "I'm going to take care of you and my baby. Don't worry about anything. I'll be home in a bit."

Somehow my parents found out. My dad said, "I made an appointment for you to go to the doctor."

"Okay," I said. I wasn't going to play stupid. I didn't want to get into a head thing with him.

The doctor called the next day with the results—positive.

My parents sat me down and said, "Do you want to keep the baby?"

"Yes," I said. I don't believe in abortion. I'd be too guilty. I feel bad about things I did when I was seven years old.

"This is what's going to happen," they told me.

I *would* cooperate with them. I had to go live with my aunt and uncle in Texas. If I didn't, I'd have to go live with my friends. They'd just put a warrant out for my arrest as a missing person. Then they'd take my baby, because they would prove that I was incompetent.

"I'm not going to get into more trouble," I thought

to myself. "I don't need a police record. I'll just do as they say."

A week after that, I moved. That's three months ago.

Now I'm five months, two weeks, and six days pregnant. My Uncle Joe is a fancy stockbroker. He's not around much. My Aunt Helene is a teacher. She runs things. Things have to be *her* way.

At first, I told her I didn't feel her rules applied to me. Number one, I wasn't her child. Number two, I wasn't going to be living under any roof with rules.

I mean, their house has roaches. I'd never seen a roach in my life until I moved in with them. They put me in a pink bedroom. Damn it, pink is not my color. They said I had a twenty-minute phone limit. How can anybody abide by that rule? I feel like I'm living in a rehab. Yech!

I have to see a therapist. I have to keep up with my prenatal doctor's appointments, checkups. I was fourteen weeks when I went for my first one. And I have to go to this school with other pregnant girls. I'm in ninth grade.

Before this, I had never been around pregnant people in my life. It's awkward.

Some of the girls are nice. A lot of them are two-faced. One is black and Mexican, and she thinks she's white. Another one is white and, to me, she's deranged. She's always talking about how her boyfriend tried to kill her in front of everybody at the mall.

A while ago, I got another phone call from Darrell. He tried to play games. He said, "I realized I'm not ready for the responsibility. Anyway, you're too young. Why don't you give it up?"

"No," I told him. "I have some money. I have the will. If you're not ready, I can't force you. If you want to do something, you will."

I decide being rebellious isn't working. I'm just messing up, trying to test people. I back down with my aunt.

The therapist wants me to talk about how I feel being adopted. "I was four months old," I tell her. "I know nothing about my birth parents. I don't think about them much, but when I do, it kind of bothers me."

I'd rather concentrate on my grades. I've been keeping them up. When I do that, my aunt rewards me. She lets me do what I want. My teachers seem to do that, too.

They even watch out for who we date. They don't want anyone around who'll pull us down. They focus on how we should treat our child properly, cooperate with other people, and if we have an attitude problem, change it.

We all have to work in day care and take parenting classes. I don't feel as nervous about kids any more. Except newborns, I can't stand newborns. Other than that, I'm fine.

After the baby's born, I'll stay here with my relatives for a while. I can't live with my parents, and they won't consent to my living anywhere else.

I'll tell you one thing, though. My child is not going to fuck up. I'm going to make sure of it. I'm going to be strict with my child, very strict.

I'm going to set rules and she has to follow them. If she doesn't, she won't get rewarded. Beyond that, I'll figure it out when the time comes. I understand kids.

LATISU MUNIRAH, PH.D., COORDINATOR, PREGNANT AND PARENTING ADDICTS RECOVERY PROGRAM, HAIGHT-ASHBURY FREE CLINIC, SAN FRANCISCO

Women often are involved with drugs because of a man. Their partner turns them on to it. How do you say "no" to this person you're with both emotionally and physically?

You ignore that he hasn't fulfilled his dreams. He doesn't feel good about himself. And then you lose sight of your own goals. You chase the drug.

When you do drugs, you skip over parts of your life. You miss the natural experiences of growing up. If you're already a mother and you're doing drugs, there's less time being spent on the needs of your child.

When adults speak to teenagers, you don't listen much. But what you could do is find another teenager who's been there. Ask about drugs and pregnancy, drugs and parenting. What are the effects for her and her children?

Then talk to people in recovery from substance abuse. Find out what kind of changes they had to make in their lives. How did they set limits on friends as well as themselves? How did they learn to say, "You can't be using around me."

Stop using drugs as soon as you can. Get involved in a support system. It could be just one other person.

Listen to your inner voice. You *do* have an inner voice. And listen to what adults who are totally interested in your welfare are saying. Let them help you help yourself.

"We're staying together!"

ALISON, 16 YEARS OLD

"Are you a virgin?" Bobby asked me on our first date. We had skipped school and spent the whole day together. Right away I felt like I knew him all my life, but just never came in contact with him.

"No," I said, wishing that wasn't the answer.

"Well, how come you didn't wait?" he said, 'cause he had.

"If I could change my past, I would. It's something you're going to have to live with."

We asked each other more questions. What his life and my life were like.

Bobby was beat a lot. His dad was an alcoholic. I told him I was sort of a party animal, into drinking. And I did try drugs. He said, "You don't need to get drunk or high. If I ever catch you, that's the end."

I told him how my parents believed in the belt, too, and I didn't. I was only allowed out once a weekend, Saturday until 11:00 P.M. even if I behaved.

They were afraid of me getting pregnant. "I won't," I said.

Bobby had a twenty-three-year-old sister with two divorces, two kids, and no money. He didn't want that to happen to him.

On prom night, a couple months after our first date,

we took a back road home and talked about sex. "We're not going to do anything until we have protection," he said.

I'd never used anything before. I even had a close call where my period didn't come for three months. I didn't expect to hear that. Most guys are pushy. I'd never waited like this. It felt different.

Bobby even went with me to Planned Parenthood for the pills.

Three days later, my dad picked me up after my job. When I was in the bank cashing my check, he went through my purse. He found them. Well, he threw a fit.

"Would you rather have me not use anything?" I asked him.

"It's not right," he said. "I'm ashamed of you."

My ma told me it was hard to accept that I didn't go to her.

"I was scared," I said. "We never really talked about sex. I didn't want you to forbid me from seeing Bobby."

Bobby didn't come over for a while after that. Then he came over, but stayed outside and honked. Finally, I persuaded him to come in. He thought they'd hate him, thinking he forced me into doing something. But really, it was both of our choices.

My dad said, "You can only see Bobby once a weekend—here. We're doing this for your own good."

"You don't understand," I said. "I'm really hurting. You're taking away something that I really care about." Me and Bobby wanted to be alone.

They would yell. I wouldn't. I was too busy crying.

My parents figured if I didn't have the pills, I wouldn't have sex. They figured wrong.

I had a year's prescription. My dad had only taken one month's supply. When I ran out, I never went back to get more. I didn't tell Bobby. There were a couple times I'd forgotten to take a pill. I thought we were careful enough.

Maybe two months later, though, I had signs. I was late. My breasts hurt bad. I had to go to the bathroom a lot.

What am I going to do? was my first thought.

I went to the health department to get a pregnancy test. It came back negative. I was confused. Maybe all those signs were nerves. I was upset. I took some pamphlets on teen pregnancy. I didn't know anything.

On New Year's, my ma asked, "Are you pregnant?"

"No," I told her, since my test had been negative. Two weeks later, I took a home pregnancy test. Positive. I didn't know what happened with that first one. The doctor said, "Sometimes there's a mistake."

I was alone when I took it. I knew there was no reason to be sad. Bobby would always be there for me. When I told him, he was happy. He knew he had to take on the responsibility. And he was willing to do that. He'd get a job.

We were both scared of telling our parents. We didn't want them to hate us. Finally, I told his ma. She told his dad.

"Well, look what mess you got into now," his dad said to him. "Your ma and me were too young, too. We never had a good life. We never went to college. We didn't want that to happen to you."

Bobby told him not to worry. I was going to take a year off after I had the baby. Then I was going to sign up for college.

I first let my dad know over the phone. I reminded him that Ma was nineteen when she had me. And my gramma was seventeen when she had her first child. I could handle it.

I'm about six months pregnant now. As soon as I met Bobby, I started gaining weight. He took me to eat all the time. I went from a skinny 100 pounds to 120. What with being pregnant, now I weigh 146.

I may look like an oversized balloon, but Bobby still loves me. He tells me that all the time. He's given me everything I've ever wanted—not just buying me things, either. He really shows me that he cares.

	WATCH WHAT YOU EAT[5]
◯	What a pregnant woman eats can set up a child for a lifetime of allergies. During pregnancy, some of the foods you may have to cut out are eggs, red meat, and dairy products.

Like, I try to eat real good. I eat breakfast every morning, usually a bowl of cereal. A hot lunch at school. Then I eat supper. Usually I like to have a snack. And Twinkies are my favorite.

Usually Bobby will buy me a can of fruit. But yesterday he knew I felt uncomfortable. He bought me a bunch of Twinkies and hid them in my locker. I thought it was cute.

I love spinach. Now I can't even look at it. I can't have salt, either. I can't have pop, because there's salt in it. My blood pressure is up. I've had swelling in my feet, ankles, and legs. It's hard for me to bend over.

The doctor says, "You hold a lot of water in your body." He's afraid of toxemia. He never explains what that means. He just says it's when the baby is in an icky environment. If I get it, they have to do an emergency C-section. That's where they cut you open and take out the baby.

Last Sunday night, the baby didn't move. The next morning it still didn't move. I got scared. I went to the doctor's office, but he found the heartbeat. It was strong. He said, "Babies are like people. They have days when they like to be lazy. Don't worry."

All my family pats my belly and says, "Boy, you're getting big." I think it's brought me and my ma closer. My dad's more understanding, too.

I feel like I've grown up a lot. I'm taking things more seriously. Every penny I get now usually goes towards the baby.

I didn't think it would cost as much. I'm getting most of my things used, but it still adds up. We got a cradle. That was fifty dollars, brand new. We got a crib, five dollars, used. We have to get a stroller, a car seat, a high chair. We need a ton of clothes, like sleepers and stuff.

But me and Bobby are not taking it fast. We're not getting married. We're getting engaged. We won't get married until we both know what we want to do.

He has a part-time job now that pays a hundred dollars a week. Once it's summer, he can work full time. We don't know what kinds of problems we'll face. But we agreed, if something happens, we'll talk it out.

After the baby's born, I'm going to ask my parents whether Bobby can stay here weekends. I'll give him my room. I'll sleep downstairs on the couch. He wants to be part of it. He wants to wake up with the baby.

If they say no, I'll probably stay at his house on the weekends. Let him get up and feed the baby. He can't during the week, because he has school and work.

I'm going to get a job, too. My ma already told me she'll watch the baby. Of course, I'll pay her. I'll be living at home. I'll have a full-time job until I go to college. Then I'll have a part-time job. And if my mother goes back to work, Bobby's ma said she can help.

It's funny. This started out about love and sex. Now that I'm pregnant, we don't do it that much. I never feel like having sex anymore. It hurts. Bobby's understanding.

You know, I'm happy about being pregnant and everything. My girlfriends are happy, too. They consider themselves aunties. They know that me and Bobby will never break up. Still…there were things that I wanted to do. I wish I would have waited.

BILL CANNON, YOUNG FATHERS COUNSELOR,

THE DOOR, NEW YORK CITY

I work with young fathers. Generally when it's still a pregnancy, you want to be involved. What happens between then and when the baby arrives—that's a different story.

I try to help expectant fathers realize this pregnancy is a *big thing*. It's going to change your life. And being told you're going to be a father produces anxiety. Inside you feel stress. Outside, though, you're, "Hey, it's cool. Let's swing with it."

If you're in this situation, and you come to me, I say, "Let's talk about what your life is like now." I try to get you to think about how you'd be if your girlfriend wasn't pregnant.

"What's your home life like?" I ask. "What kind of relationship do you have with your father? Are you in school? How are you doing? What are your plans for the future?"

Once you get a handle on that, you should think about how your life might change if you become a father.

There's no storybook father, no storybook family relationship. You don't automatically end up with 3.2 kids in a home in suburbia with a backyard and a dog. You have to look at your life squarely. How can you put things together to be the *best* father possible?

What comes up a lot is this: how can you understand

what it is to be a father when you never really knew your own dad? Maybe you're in the same situation he was. And you definitely have some feelings about that!

You know what his absence has meant to you. You might not be able to talk about it, but the anger you feel translates into your not wanting your kids to grow up like that.

You should think, "What kind of father do I want to be?"

Maybe you say, "I'm going to be there for my kids. I'm going to do things with them. I'm going to talk to them when they have problems."

You've got this child on the way. You want to do the right thing. You've explored what your life is like. Now let's talk about how we can merge that. What are your options?

For starters, how are you going to support that child? You tell me you quit school. You've got to find a job. And you're thinking about dealing drugs.

Well, if you deal, there's a strong possibility you'll wind up either in jail or dead. If that happens, you take yourself *away* from the child you want to have a life with.

If you're sitting in my office, I tell you that.

What I hear is, "Okay, I won't deal drugs. But, man, come on, minimum wage at Burger King?!"

At this point, though, you don't have the skills to get a better-paying job. That's reality. If you want to be involved with your son or daughter, you have to work at minimum wage...for now.

This doesn't mean you have to do it for the rest of your life. Organizations like the one I work for can help you, or you can help yourself get back into school or take the GED. There is a future.

Maybe the idea of working for minimum wage makes you mad. But you made the decision to have this child, which means that it's no longer entirely about you. Now a major part of your time is spent preparing for your child to live in this world. You have to start accepting that you are responsible for that individual.

A good father begins *now* to look to the future. You do things that will ensure that the child will eat, grow, and develop in as healthy a way as possible.

I won't put down a set standard. Each of you has to consider your own situation. A good father in many cases is someone who's doing the best that he can. He's trying regardless of obstacles.

It's hard being a male in our society. We are raised and socialized to be screwed up in how to interact with the world around us, and particularly with our female partners.

And, generally, males feel that part of what defines our manhood is *fathering* children. Just because we don't have a job, or we don't have a stable family support system, or the future is unclear, that will not necessarily keep us from fulfilling that aspect of our manhood.

In fact, if all those other things aren't in place, if we're feeling low self-esteem because we can't find a job, because we're not doing well in school, we may look to fathering a child as the one thing that will establish our manhood.

I have a theory. I think that fathering children at a young age—particularly among so-called minorities—is a survival mechanism. Not only survival as an individual, but survival as a people.

On a certain level you know that things are *not* great for African-American people, for a lot of Latino people. I do believe that part of what's happening is a sense of realizing that these communities are in danger of being wiped out.

I hear a lot, "My fucking girlfriend's driving me crazy!" You feel that part of being a good father means being a good partner. Well, that's not always the same thing.

If your relationship with your girl doesn't work out, that happens. That does *not* mean right then and there you break off your relationship with your son or daughter. Instead, for however long you can, you should be involved in the development of your child.

55

PREGNANCY

GARY, 17 YEARS OLD

"YOU AIN'T KILLING MY KID!"

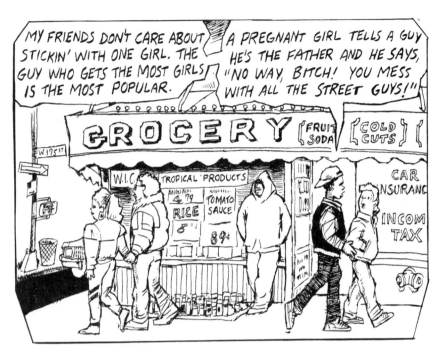

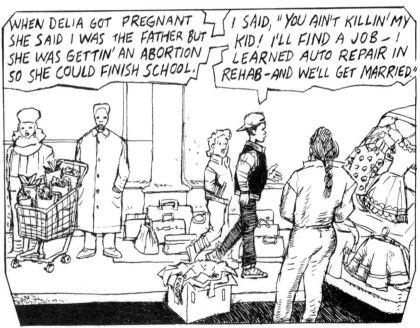

SHE GOT THIS KOOL-AID SMILE ON HER FACE AND SAID, "YES." I MOVED IN WITH HER TO HER AUNT'S APARTMENT.

HER AUNT'S FRIEND USED DRUGS AND THEY KEPT FIGHTING WITH US. ONE DAY HER AUNT SCREAMED AT US, "GET OUT!"

DRESS SALON — CHILDREN — BEAUT

CORSETS — STROLLER SALE — NAIL TIPS

WE WENT TO A SHELTER. THEY SAID 16 WAS TOO YOUNG TO STAY THERE. WE SLEPT AT DIFFERENT PEOPLE'S APARTMENTS.

BUT DELIA CRIED EVERY NIGHT. SHE MISSED HER AUNT. FINALLY, SHE WENT BACK HOME.

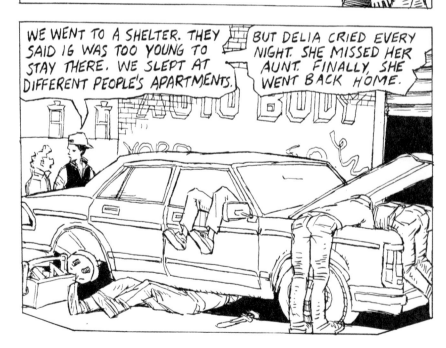

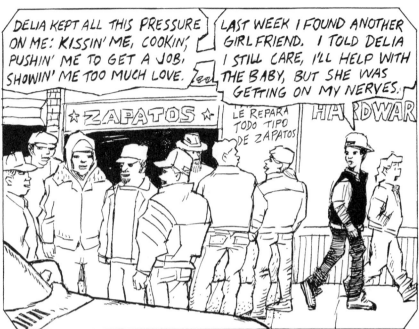

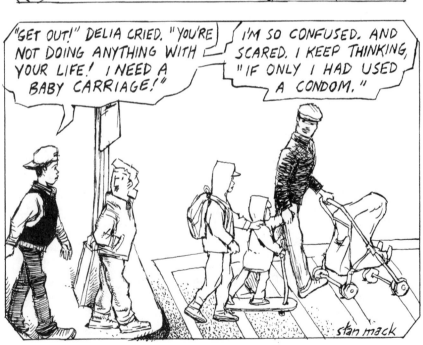

JANIE GORE GOLAN, M.S.W., PRINCIPAL

INVESTIGATOR, STUDY OF INFANTS AND CHILDREN

PRENATALLY EXPOSED TO CRACK AND COCAINE,

RICHARDSON, TEXAS

When I was sixteen, I did some research in a hospital emergency room. One day a doctor said, "I want you to see this baby."

"What's the matter with her?" I asked.

"The mother was on angel dust. Her baby was born without a brain. That's called anencephalic."

The next day the baby died.

That's when I began to learn the effects of drugs on a fetus and a child.

Today, when pregnant teens come and tell us they're using marijuana, we ask if they know that smoking *any-thing* has an impact on the fetus. If they're talking about heroin or cocaine, drinking two four-packs of wine coolers a day, or even using over-the-counter drugs like diet pills, that's all going to affect the fetus.

Put simply, you take something into your body. It goes to your bloodstream. And it also goes on a direct line to a fetus. A drug that speeds up your heartbeat is going to speed up the heartbeat of a fetus. A drug that hurts you is going to hurt the fetus. The reaction is almost immediate.

The fetus is developing every step of the way. Every single day, something new occurs. We know that the baby's heart, lungs, liver, kidneys—all its vital organs are formed during the first trimester, the first twelve weeks of pregnancy. The limbs are formed, too.

We know that any type of drug, with the probable exception of those prescribed by a doctor, *may* adversely affect that growth. Kids may be born with too small or too large a head, microcephalic or macrocephalic. They can be born with one eye higher than the other. They can be missing arms or legs. They can be born without kidneys. They can develop cerebral palsy.

Children whose mothers drink during the pregnancy can be born with what's called fetal alcohol syndrome, FAS. You look at a child with FAS, you see the eyes are very small. The child appears to be sullen. The children might also be mentally retarded.

With two to three drinks a day, a pregnant woman increases by 11 percent the chances of giving birth to a child with FAS. Four or more drinks, it's 19 percent. The more you drink, the greater the danger.

When you use crack or cocaine during a pregnancy, the child you give birth to may at first look fine, healthy and normal. Then a week later, he or she could have the shakes and be irritable. And by irritable, I mean screaming and not able to sleep. Crack babies don't tolerate feedings well. They are extemely demanding.

As they grow older and you hug them, they won't hug back. Instead, they go rigid or act like a wet doll. They are not able to respond or give love in return. There's no comforting these children. Some can't sit still and they have high energy.

Some medical professionals say, "The fetus isn't affected by crack or cocaine. It's poverty which causes these problems. When these children are born, get them into the right environment and they'll be fine."

One thing, though, you can't forget. Doing drugs during a pregnancy is *not* going to *help* you or your child. If you're using drugs, see a doctor. Level with him or her. That person will hopefully be able to get you the kind of help you need. You can still increase the opportunities for your child.

"I want a baby."

KARA, 19 YEARS OLD

When I was seventeen, in the twelfth grade, my family moved away. My mother and I didn't get along, and I was left behind. I was shocked.

I had a $1.23, a blanket, a teddy bear, and an old key to the house.

I spent that first week there, in our house, until the new people moved in. Then the nurse at school found out. She wanted to send me to a group home.

"*No*," I told her.

"Well, I'm sorry," she said, "but you can't come to school if you don't have a parent in the area."

I'd be with friends in the day and sleep in the park at night. I was really frightened. Nobody around. Cold and dark. Sprinklers going on and off at two in the morning. It seemed like I was being watched.

Before this, I'd always had a room of my own.

But I'd also been raised never to give up. I figured, "It can't be like this forever. How can I get out of this situation?" When I tried to sign up for an adult education program, I found out about the Job Corps. I could live on a campus, take classes, and get my GED.

On my eighteenth birthday, I start the Job Corps and meet this guy, Randy. I'm in love. Randy takes me to meet his family—his mom, his dad, his sisters and their children.

They're homeless and live in a motel. I'm, "Ohmigosh, I've never experienced anything like this." They invite me to move in. One week, we only have potato chips for dinner.

I don't care where I am. It's like, I'm with this guy. I love him. He loves me. We're here together. That's all I need.

Randy got a job driving a truck and I was a manager at Burger King. But still we never had enough money for first and last months' rent. That's what you need to rent an apartment.

One day I called work, told them I felt *terrible*. The boss said, "Oh, you just don't want to come in."

"I'm not faking," I said. "I'm in pain."

Finally, it got so bad that Randy took me to the emergency room. They said, "You're staying overnight. You're pregnant."

I had what's called a tubal pregnancy. The fetus was stuck in the tube, not in the uterus where it's supposed to be. They told me if I waited another week, the fetus would have grown and made the tube explode. I could have died! I was trembling.

I hadn't wanted to be pregnant. But then, afterwards,

it was, "Gosh, I lost my baby." Pretty soon, we wanted to have a child. We'd get married and everything.

We tried and tried and tried. We went to three different doctors. They told me I had a hormone deficiency. Forget about having kids.

I was going through deep depression. I was beating up Randy, saying, "It's all your fault."

He didn't deserve it. He'd say, "I'm sorry, but it's not me. It's not me."

It was hard to accept that I couldn't have children. I mean, that's why I started working at Burger King. I wanted to be somewhere I could see lots of kids—make a smile on their faces. I worked birthday parties. I saved toys and showed up with a bagful.

I'd been getting sick and had missed a period. But it didn't hit me. I'd missed a period before. I went to Planned Parenthood and they checked it out. "You're eight weeks pregnant," they told me.

I was so happy. I was jumping up and down. People were looking at me. They were sitting there, thinking, "Please, *no, no, no*, I don't want to be pregnant."

I was, like, "Yes, please, let me be pregnant." It was a great moment for me.

I called Randy and he said, "Let's get married."

"I don't know," I said. "Maybe we should wait. We need to find some place to live—on our own."

But we still couldn't afford rent.

Randy stayed on with his family. I went to a homeless shelter. It was not for pregnant people. And I was the youngest person there. There were both men and women, men downstairs and women upstairs. You had to be out by nine in the morning and you couldn't come back until five thirty.

When I talked to a case worker, she said, "We should look for a place you can get the support you need."

That's when I came to this place, Florence Crittenton

Services. I'm the oldest one living here. But at least I get the backup help and health services I need. I've been here two months and I think it's great.

In fact, I don't know where I'd be if I wasn't here. Randy can't take care of me. And I'm not interested in marriage. Here, they're making me look in the right direction.

I don't want to live the way we lived. I don't want my child to live that way, either. Randy and I are growing distant.

I'm going to college now, taking a couple of courses. My favorite is the psychology of stress. I walk in here and I see the total amount of stress in all the girls. What I'm learning helps me understand.

I'm sharing a room. Once you've been at Florence Crittenton three months, they say you can get a room of your own. I had seven roommates at the homeless shelter. Here I just have one.

That's enough, considering the mood changes I'm going through. When you're pregnant, your moods go up and down. I used to have patience. Lately, I get so frustrated.

A lot of the girls say, "Oh, this food is nasty. It's cold and stale." They don't know what gross food is. They say, "Gee, when I turn eighteen, I'm out of here." They don't know what real life is. I try to tell them it isn't easy.

I tell them, they can't give up. Help is there. They just have to look. I go to parenting classes and they should, too.

I've been around children. In the motel I helped raise Randy's sister's daughter. I've been through teething, diapers, rashes, baths. I look at it as more experience.

If I had one wish right now, I'd wish I could stay at Florence Crittenton after my baby's born. But since I'm here voluntarily and I'm over eighteen, I have to leave after the birth. It's their policy.

I have some friends who say, "Oh, I can't wait until you have a baby." So I do have places to go after this—until I get on my feet.

PART III

Abortion

PAULA WENDT, B.S., R.N., CLINIC DIRECTOR,

MEADOWBROOK WOMEN'S CLINIC,

MINNEAPOLIS, MINNESOTA

Most teenagers know that abortions are legal. They have been since 1973. But you don't know that the majority of states now have what's called either a parental consent law or a parental notice law. These both mean you first have to go to your parents and tell them you want to have an abortion.

If you don't want to tell one or both parents, there is a judicial bypass. That means you make an appointment to appear before a judge who, after hearing your situation, usually signs a petition saying you can have the abortion without a parent knowing.

As soon as you think you might be pregnant, confide in someone. Then you've got two heads working on it, instead of just one. You need somebody who's going to say to you, *We have to find out the facts right away.*

Some of you say, "But I can't tell anyone I might be pregnant, that I want an abortion."

Personally, I think this is the kind of life event that you need to share with others. And once you start sharing, you get a lot of support. Usually, you end up telling someone who's had an abortion or knows somebody who had an abortion.

I hear all the time, "I told my friend Mary I was preg-

WILL ABORTION REMAIN LEGAL?

As this book goes to press, abortion is legal in the United States. Whether that will remain true is in doubt. In 1991 the Supreme Court ruled that health care workers in clinics receiving federal government money can no longer mention abortion as a resolution to an unwanted pregnancy. If asked about the procedure, rather than offer information about all of a woman's medical options, they must answer, "We do not consider abortion an appropriate method of family planning."

State laws are changing. Some states say teenagers can make the decision to have an abortion on their own. Others require you to involve a parent or close family member in that choice.

By the time you read this chapter, the Supreme Court may have overturned what is known as *Roe* v. *Wade*, the ruling that gave women across the country the right to chose to have an abortion. For the latest information about what's legal and what's not regarding abortion in your home state, call the Planned Parenthood listed in your phone directory and/or call the toll-free hotlines of the National Abortion Federation: 1-800-772-9100 (in Washington, D.C., 667-5881).

nant and maybe going to have an abortion. Mary said, 'Well, I was never going to tell you this, but....'"

I'd like you to know that often parents are okay people to tell. Yes, you hear, "I'm hurt to learn this. I'm disappointed." But next you hear, "I love you. Your well-being is my priority. I want to help you."

I've also met parents who say to their daughter, "You little tramp, now that I know you're pregnant, you're never going to see that boyfriend again!"

You can have an abortion without telling your parents. But you never forget that you did it. Do you want to have that be a secret until you're twenty-five or thirty and decide to share it with your mom?

What you might hear then is, "Didn't you love me enough to tell me?"

You answer, "That's *exactly* why I didn't tell you. I loved you so much."

And parents have a hard time with that. Then again, there are some parents who should *never* know. You know your parents better than any counselor. After discussing it with an adult you trust, you make the judgment whether to go to them.

If there's a chance you're pregnant, buy an at-home pregnancy test. For ten or fifteen dollars, you can test yourself when nobody's around. Then call a Planned Parenthood or a women's health clinic with a medical staff and go in for pregnancy testing and decision counseling.

You want to start thinking and talking about all your options in a pregnancy. How do you see your life and your future if you continue the pregnancy and parent the child? What if you continue the pregnancy and arrange for an adoption?

Only after those conversations do we talk about abortion. By this time, most of you say, "I always thought abortion was okay. I just never thought it would happen to me."

Some of you only had sex once, and now you're pregnant. You feel caught and punished. It's hard to have to deal with all this. You feel you're being blamed for something you hardly even did.

Some of you ask, "If I have an abortion, will I go to hell?"

What I say is this: "I talk to a lot of women about that. Most say they feel God is forgiving. He understands that sometimes women need to do this."

Others say, "My parents will kill me if they find out

I'm pregnant. But I believe if I have an abortion, God will never forgive me."

"Then you must not have the abortion," I say. "To pay that kind of eternal, moral price is more than anybody should ever do."

Still others say, "I want to have the abortion, but I don't believe in them."

Nobody believes in abortion. Nobody believes that women should sometimes be made to have abortions. But we also don't believe that women should sometimes be made to have babies that they don't want and don't love.

All of us wish abortion didn't exist. It's not like people who are pro-choice think that all pregnant women should have abortions.

We think that until there is better birth control and more teaching of sex education and relationship information, we have the right to offer the option of abortion to the pregnant woman.

The former Surgeon General of the United States, C. Everett Koop, made a study and reported that abortion is a very safe procedure, both emotionally and physically. He says he tried to find out where it's dangerous and damaging. He couldn't.

That's not to say there aren't some women who regret their decision. There are some women who become depressed and even need treatment. There are some women who become suicidal because of this and other factors. And there are complications that can occur.

If you ask me, "Is an abortion totally safe?" I say, "This is like any other medical procedure. There are things that can go wrong. Perforation of the uterus, hemorrhage, all the complications associated with full-term pregnancy and labor occur here, too—only less frequently."

You have to decide for yourself, How do I feel about having an abortion?

Most women have some mixed feelings. You wonder some about what that child would have been like had it gone to term. But most women do FINE.

I also tell women of all ages, "Look, you can let somebody else make this decision. You can blame it on your mom. Blame it on your boyfriend. Blame it on us. But in the end, you're going to need to come to terms with it."

Nobody can make you go into that room and have the abortion. Some women cry, "I have no choice."

I say, "You *always* have a choice. You're in a bad situation and it looks like this is the way out for you. But you still have a choice. You can still walk out of here and stay pregnant. I will refer you to people who will help you do this."

We don't want to do abortions on women who are going to regret it.

What advice do I have for teen males involved with a pregnancy? Let's say, she's just told you, "I think I'm pregnant."

What I've seen is that the couple does better if you remain kind of neutral. You hold back a little and give her some time.

If you say, "I want you to have the abortion," she may feel you don't love her and won't love your child.

If you say, "I want you to have the baby," she may feel you want to trap her into being with you forever.

What seems to work is if you say to her, "Okay, let's talk. Tell me how you feel about this pregnancy? What are you thinking? What do you feel would be the best decision for you?"

And, at a certain point, when she says, "What's the best decision for *you*," you should say how you feel and what you're willing to do to provide. You must be honest.

Planned Parenthood has a wonderful slogan: Every child wanted. That's our goal, too.

"The best solution was abortion."

AMY, 14 YEARS OLD

I've had responsibility my whole life. My father's an alcoholic. Starting when I was six years old, I had to take care of him. I basically lived in a barroom.

I remember fourth grade most of all. We would get up in the morning about seven o'clock. I'd go to school. When I got home, I'd go down and help him in the barn. He's a farmer.

Then we'd go back up to the house, get changed, and we'd go out to a bar. We'd be there from—ooh, geeze, he got off work about six. We'd be in the bar from seven until three, four in the morning.

I drag him out to the car when the bar closes. Get him in. Most of the time, I drive him home because he's too drunk to even see. I get him home by five in the morning and get him up by seven o'clock, two hours later.

It was that way every day. On weekends, forget it, twenty-four hours in the bar. It was amazing.

I had the responsibility of cleaning the house, cooking for my father, and taking care of him, too. When he was sick, I stayed home and did his chores. I missed fifty-three days of school that year.

I met Mark when I was in eighth grade. He's older.

I liked being held, but I never really enjoyed the other part. He said he'd pull out just before he came. That way I wouldn't get pregnant.

It didn't work.

I talked to my best girlfriend. I talked to the school nurse. She said in California I didn't need a parent's permission to have an abortion. Why should I tell my dad? He barely knows I'm here. My mom left when I was little.

On a Tuesday, my girlfriend and I both cut school. She went with me for my abortion. I sat at a desk and they ask you, "Is this your first abortion?" Then you have to fill out a questionnaire. It asks about your medical history, about your periods, and things like that. They go over that with you, to double-check everything.

Next they ask you, "Are you doing this of your own free will?" They make you write it on the bottom of that paper. You have to sign it, too.

When I was back in the waiting room, all of a sudden, you could hear these voices outside *screaming*. "Don't kill your baby! Come out with us. We'll take care of you. Those people only want your money. They don't care about you. They're trying to ruin your life!"

They were pounding on the door, shoving fliers under it.

Some of the girls started crying. I got angry. I wanted a future! Were they going to help me take care of my father and a baby? At fourteen?

I was brought up a fighter. I learned how to deal with problems. For me, the best solution was abortion.

The people at the clinic took us all into a room away from the noise. Nobody left. We all stayed to have the abortion.

I had this exam so they could see how far along I was. I was two months. You sit there until this guy takes blood from you. After all that, you put on a blue gown and these funny blue shoes. This lady at a desk takes your blood pressure. Then they send you to this other room where you watch TV until you're called.

They ask you how you want them to do it. You can be asleep or they can deaden you from the hips down. I wanted to be asleep. They put you in the room where they do it. They were really nice. They stuck this needle in my wrist...the stuff that makes you go to sleep.

I was talking and they were talking. The next thing I knew, I was in the recovery room. It was over. They came and told me where I was.

You stay in the recovery room until you feel better. After about ten minutes, they let you get up and you walk around a little. They give you this pad, a Kotex, to put on for the bleeding. They had juice, graham crackers, and Tylenol for the pain. But I didn't take it.

They remind you, you shouldn't do a lot of exercising for two weeks, including no sex. I told them, "No problem."

KAREN AND BILL BELL, PARENTS OF BECKY BELL

INDIANAPOLIS, INDIANA

Karen Bell

There's an old saying, "Boys will be boys, but girls will be punished." And our daughter, Becky, paid the price. On a Friday just after her seventeenth birthday, she died from an illegal abortion.

We were going to say that Becky died of pneumonia. (On her autopsy, it says septic abortion *with* pneumonia.) At the funeral, our minister came and knelt down before us with all our friends from the community—three hundred, four hundred people.

He said, "Tell people what really happened."

As my son closed the casket, he said, "No one will ever hurt my sister again."

I had a hard time talking about sex with my daughter and my son. It was embarrassing for us. I thought, "Oh, that's like encouraging them to have sex." Parents don't want to think about that.

But we *did* talk about it. I'd say, "Beck, honey, if you ever do anything, please protect yourself."

I never even mentioned abortion. That kind of thing wouldn't happen to us. I had my girl and my boy, the *perfect* family. I was home every day with my kids. And they were almost grown.

	POST-ABORTION DANGER SIGNS[3]
○	After an abortion, immediately contact the provider if you have any of these symptoms: severe pain; chills or fever with a temperature of 100.4°F (38°C) or more; bleeding that saturates more than one sanitary pad an hour; foul-smelling discharge from your vagina; continuing symptoms of pregnancy.

Becky was a junior. She was a horseback rider, an animal lover. She was in the band. She played the flute. She was such an easy, gentle child. She wouldn't hurt anything or anyone. Except herself.

Well, she went out a few times with this guy, a family friend, supposedly. He told her he was sterile. He'd had the mumps. She believed him. When she discovered she was pregnant, she told him. He said these very words, "Get the hell out of my life."

She went to Planned Parenthood. We talked to the counselor she talked to. She told us what Beck said: she loved us and was so ashamed of herself. "How can I go to my parents, say I've had sex, let alone that I'm pregnant? And then on top of it, I want an abortion?"

Becky said, "I won't hurt my mom and dad. I don't want to disappoint them. I just won't tell them."

That's when the counselor explained that in Indiana—like lots of states—if you're under eighteen, you need permission from a parent to have an abortion. The only other choice was to go to a judge in Indianapolis and petition the courts.

But Beck knew this particular judge's reputation. He was against abortion. Going to him was a waste of time. Anyway, if she couldn't tell her mom and dad, how could she stand before a stranger and beg for a waiver of the law? And how could she get out of school without us being contacted?

It would be terrifying. She didn't even know how to get downtown alone.

Becky was desperate. One option she had was to cross the state line to Kentucky. It's a hundred miles away. In that state, though, you don't need a parent's permission to get an abortion. It's safe and legal there. But she would have had to figure out how to get away from home for a couple days, arrange for a car, and find the money to pay for it.

How do you explain that to a parent?

I remember how sad she was on her birthday. She had tears in her eyes. I said, "Honey, be happy. You've got everything to live for."

A few days later, she said she was going to a party on the south side of town. There was a girl in trouble she wanted to be with and make happy. We didn't know then that the girl was Becky herself.

They've never found who did it to Becky. But something dirty was introduced into her body. She came home sick that night. We doctored her. She got up the next day with a stiff neck. She went to work and then to school on Monday.

After that, we doctored her for the flu. We kept saying, "You're going to the doctor." She would not go. She didn't bleed or anything until Friday. She started to hemorrhage.

She smiled and said, "Mommy, I started my *period*. Help me to the bathroom." We had to carry her.

Bill said, "She's going to the hospital."

Becky was so relieved. She thought in her heart that she was safe. The pregnancy was over. The last thing she said was, "Mommy and Dad, I love you." Then she gave us her little ring off her hand.

She died that way.

If Beck had come to us and said, "I'm pregnant," I'm going to tell you the truth. I would have been furious. I probably would have said, "You've ruined yourself. What will people think?" We live in this community that I care about.

But the choice would have been hers. If she wanted an abortion, if she wanted to keep the baby, whatever. But we didn't get the chance to tell her.

Bill Bell

Here's my plea. Maybe there's a young woman reading this book that's desperate and in trouble. Please don't do what our daughter did.

Tell your parents what's happening. There's no safer place, no better care and guidance than what you'll get from your parents. I say that with this exception: Not every family is a loving one.

Still, you're in a race against time. Once you find yourself pregnant, you have to analyze your particular family situation. You have to find out what you're faced with in the state where you live. The state laws are different.

I encourage you to seek the advice of adults. If you feel you can't go to your parents, it's still so important that you get a mature adult involved for some guidance and counseling.

I can only think if Becky had gone to a friend of the family, a school counselor, that someone could have, would have, helped her make better decisions. Don't, please don't, get an *illegal* abortion. And don't try to take something or do something to abort yourself.

Karen Bell

I wonder, "How did this parental consent law help us? How did it help Becky?" I envy every parent and child who can put their arms around each other tonight.

I'm against abortion.

I work as a volunteer at a pregnancy center. We're listed under "Clinics" in the yellow pages of the telephone
directory. Girls call up and want to know information
about abortions. They ask how much an abortion costs. Do
we perform them?

We say, "We don't perform abortions here in the
office."

You see, our goal is to persuade you *not* to have an
abortion. If you knew ahead of time that was our goal, you
might not come in. Across the country, there are places like
us with the same purpose and methods.

Once you're here, we give you a pregnancy test, show
you videos about the issue, and find out why you want an
abortion. Often we hear, "My parents will freak." Or "It
will screw up my life." Or "I don't have the money." For
most girls, though, the reason is that having a baby is
inconvenient.

You want to deny you're pregnant. We say, "Imagine
you wanted to be pregnant. You were happily married and
had lots of money. You'd go, 'Yippee, I have a baby growing inside me.' It's just that today the circumstances are different. You can't, though, deny a baby is there."

If you have any religious background, we remind you
that God says it's wrong to murder. And abortion is mur-

dering a baby. You also face medical and psychological risks.

We know mostly you're scared. This is an upheaval to your life. We don't promise you any quick fixes. It's a lie if we say it's easy. But we can help you during and after the pregnancy through referrals to such places as prenatal clinics, drug programs, and adoption agencies.

"My mom said, 'ABORTION.'"

SHALIMAR, 15 YEARS OLD

I started crying when I told Yor-El I was pregnant. He said, "What are you crying for? It's nothing to be ashamed about. I'm happy."

We hadn't been going together long or anything, just a couple months, but I felt, "He's the person I want to spend the rest of my life with."

Pretty soon, though, I kept hearing from him, "You have to tell your mother. It's important that she know."

The next thing I knew, mature, nineteen-year-old Yor-El was saying, "Shalimar, you should live first before you tie yourself down. You shouldn't keep it." That made me want to cry more.

I thought he cared. That's what was special about him. When you saw me, you saw him. He took me to see *Exorcist III* on our first date. He gave me a Nintendo game for my birthday. We were a nice couple.

Now he was changing his mind. I shut him out. He came to see me. I just ignored him, like he wasn't there. I was hurt. Even though I'm young and hadn't lived and everything, I wanted that baby. I wanted to hear him say, "Yeah, keep it."

Instead, he called me and said, "This isn't working out. I'm not going to put my life on hold for you. We should just be friends."

Friends!? What did that mean? We were still going to

do everything together? We weren't going to see other people? But we would just be friends?

I put on some clothes and went walking to the river. Later he called back and said he was worried about me. I said, "I don't know why you're worried, if we're just friends."

"What do *you* want to do?" he said.

"I want it to be like it was before."

"Okay," he said, "but I'm not used to you acting this way. Just have the abortion and then don't think about it. If you keep it, I can't really support you."

I didn't know what to do.

My girlfriends said if they were me, they would keep it. That made it even harder. To them, to me, abortion is murder.

I cried enough tears to last a lifetime. Then Yor-El went back to saying, "Talk to your mother."

I was, like, "If I'm going to have an abortion, why tell my mom?" In New York, where I live, you can have an abortion without telling your parents.

I told my mother.

"Well, you know what you have to do," she said. I knew she was talking about abortion. I just knew. And I was mad.

"I don't want an abortion."

She said I was messing up my life. If I kept it, I had to move out of the house, go into an apartment, and get on welfare.

Think of my future, she said. What kind of life could I give a child? Didn't I see from her it was hard to be a single mother? She was moving up the ladder at work. She didn't want to quit her job to stay home and be a grandmother.

I went to talk to the school counselor. I told her I thought my mother was forcing her beliefs on me. She wasn't giving me a choice. She wasn't being supportive.

The counselor said I had a right to be angry. This *was* my decision. But, also, if I had an abortion, afterwards I had a right to grieve. About three days later, lots of girls feel real bad—emotionally. That's not God punishing us. It's just our hormones changing.

"I just want my mom to understand what I'm going through. My pain. I want Yor-El to understand...."

"I don't think the man ever understands when something like this happens," the counselor said.

That night my mom told me I had to go to a doctor. When I went, he asked me what was I going to do? I said, "I want to keep it, but I can't."

He said, "When you have children in the future, they'll be happy because you'll be able to support them. Don't worry. You have many years to still have them."

I felt I was in another world. I wanted to die. I wrote a poem, "The Decision." Here's the last part:

...I had this decision to make.
A HARD one.
How could I kill something that would resemble me?
And the man I love with all my heart?
For he was part of me.
He was part of him.
And killing it would be like killing part of us that could
  never be again.
My love for him hurt every day.
Knowing what I would have to do....

I scheduled the appointment for an abortion.

"I had to get a judge to say 'Okay' to my abortion."

HEATHER PEARSON, 20 YEARS OLD[5]

At the age of fourteen, I got very sick with bronchitis. My mom took me to the doctor. He said, "Well, we'll go have an X ray."

In the examining room there was one of those posters that read: "If you might be pregnant, let us know." All of a sudden, I remembered, "I haven't had my period!" To be honest, I hadn't even thought about pregnancy until I saw that sign.

You hear about it happening, but the girls who get pregnant are *stupid*. They're sluts. They're the ones always in trouble. I wasn't doing drugs. I wasn't out drinking. So why would I worry about getting pregnant? That's how I thought.

Of course, I wasn't using birth control, either.

"I might be pregnant," I said to the doctor. "Can I have a pregnancy test without letting my mom know?"

My mom talked about sex, but when she did, she said it was wrong. I was too young.

But for me, boys and having crushes were in the picture by second grade. By eighth grade I started going with Tim. He was a year older. I liked that he was mature and had a pretty good head on him. He was open and honest.

He was always with me. We would meet on our bikes at five in the morning. We began school at seven thirty.

Then we'd be together again after school until ten at night. This was big time stuff and his mother hated me.

I can still see it to this day. As I walked out of the doctor's office, he flashed a piece of paper. On it was the word positive. I was pregnant. I got in the car and cried.

First of all, I told Tim. He was surprised. We were both scared to death. We didn't really know what to do. I wanted to close my eyes, go to sleep, and when I woke up, this would not be happening.

Then, like anybody else, I kind of fantasized about it. "This is wonderful. A baby!" I didn't, though, go off into that world of "Oh, Tim and I will get married. We'll have this baby...." Sure I was madly in love with him and he was my first love. Still, I was fourteen years old.

I worried to myself, "How will I support this baby? Be serious. There's no way I can." My mom would have to do it.

Then there was adoption. I felt I wasn't the right type of person. If I did that, I'd still wonder today, "What is that baby doing? Are they loving parents?"

I talked to my girlfriends. One said she'd be there for me whatever I did. Another one thought babies are neat. She didn't believe in abortion, she told me.

To me, abortion was just a word. I didn't know anything more.

Tim and I agreed it was time to tell my mother. The

problem was I didn't know how. We've always been close, but she's the kind with high expectations for me and success and the future. She wasn't going to be happy.

I hated school, but to her, education is everything. She doesn't have a college degree. So even though she always had a job, like executive secretary or office manager, it was a struggle raising me and my sister.

See, she and my dad divorced when I was five. He was an alcoholic and that broke them up. I don't remember much of him around the house. After he left, I only saw him a couple times a year. He was almost a stranger.

Anyway, I called my mom at work, so I wouldn't have to look at her face. "I have something to tell you...." I said over the phone.

My mom didn't say things to make me feel worse than I already did. "What do you want to do, Heather?" she asked.

"I think I want to have an abortion," I said.

She called the Medical Women's Clinic to find out what I needed to do. When she hung up the phone, she couldn't believe it. In the state of Minnesota, before I could get an abortion, I had to tell *both* my biological parents or go to court to get a judge to say it was okay.

My mom was real mad. She was the only supporting parent. She had total custody of me and my sister. She was doing everything. She could sign for anything, but not this.

I said, "I'm not going to tell my dad."

My mom and I agreed; I'd go to court. But that frightened me more than having the abortion. It was too personal a thing to tell some judge, a complete stranger.

I thought only bad people go to court. You know, like in the movies. And I really didn't have any idea about the court process. That freaked me out. "I can't understand why we have to go to court," I told my mom. What could she do? It was the law.

The clinic schedules both the appointment for court and for the abortion. It all happens in one day. At that time, I'm sick.

I walk in a restaurant, and if there is cigarette smoke, I run to the bathroom. I can't eat certain foods. All day long, I'm nauseated.

So that morning we get up at this awful, early hour and I'm sick, as usual. Tim, my mom, and me drive to the clinic with a bucket in the car.

Once there, the three of us watch a video about what will happen that day. Then they do another pregnancy test and feel my stomach to tell how far along I am.

I talk to a nice counselor, too. We're alone. She asks me what concerns I might have. I want to know more about the procedure, the abortion. What exactly happens? Can I be put to sleep? Do they charge extra for that? Can I have somebody hold my hand? And then I ask about the pain.

"It's different for everybody," she says. "For some people, it hurts a lot. For others, it's like very strong menstrual cramps."

She wants to know how I made my decision. Am I feeling good about it? Is anybody forcing me into this? She's caring. And if I want to back out, this is my chance.

I feel comfortable with my decision. We talk about my future plans, including birth control. It's a neat session. Finally we talk about court, what will happen. By now it's about ten in the morning.

I'm starving. You can't eat after midnight. With morning sickness, if you eat dry toast, the nausea goes away. I couldn't even eat that.

And I'm so scared.

We go to court, the three of us. We sit out in a big, open hallway, a bunch of us, other girls from clinics. Anybody can walk by and know why we're there. We're waiting to see a judge to get permission for an abortion.

Our privacy has been stripped away. It's awful!

First they call you in to talk to a court-appointed attorney. She asks all these personal questions. Why do I want to have an abortion? What is my family situation? Why don't I want to tell my father? Why won't I consider adoption?

It makes me feel worse, because I'm required to tell this person, another stranger.

Next I go wait in the courtroom, where the jurors' bench is. You get called in one by one to the judge's chambers. My mom goes in with me. And you know what? All he says is, "Hi. Why do you want an abortion?"

"I don't feel I'm ready to have a child. I want to go on to school."

"Fine," he says, scribble, scribble, and I'm out of there.

Then in the afternoon, I have the abortion. The waiting room is full. Some are having abortions. Some are supportive friends and relatives.

When I get called in, there's a lady who goes in with me. She says, "Will you please strip from the waist down and we'll begin."

She's there to hold my hand and talk to me. For about thirty seconds, my mind starts racing. I think, "What am I doing here? This isn't real."

Two more people come and they start. The lady asks me questions about school, and at the same time explains to me exactly what they're doing.

She says, like, "They put the speculum in. And now they're going to give your cervix a shot. You're going to feel a little pinch." And that's just what happened.

"Now they're going to put this in and turn on a machine. You're going to feel severe cramps...." I have cramps, but they aren't bad.

Then they stop and scrape the insides of my uterus to make sure they got it all. They do this one more time and it's done. It's probably a total of five minutes.

After that, I go sit in the waiting room, have toast and juice, and a half hour later—go home.

Now it's nearly six years later. Tim and I kept seeing each other for the next year or so. Then we grew apart.

As far as the abortion, I have absolutely no regrets. Sometimes I think, wow, I would have a five-year-old! There's no way I could have done it.

What I think was awful, though, was the court experience. In a state where 50 percent of the minors are growing up in single-parent families, they say we need to tell both our parents. It's not fair.

PART IV

Foster Care

"My stepdad got me pregnant!"

STEPHANIE, 16 YEARS OLD

When I was a kid, I lived with my mother, my stepfather, my stepbrother, and my half sister. By the time I was eleven, my stepfather was coming into my bedroom and raping me. If I told anyone, he said he'd do the same thing to my little sister.

Two years later, I got pregnant. He was the father.

To deal with it, I pretended it wasn't true. By the time I was six or seven months pregnant, kids at school would say, "Stephanie, are you pregnant?"

"What?" I'd say. "Are you crazy? I've just gained weight."

Finally my mother said, "Go have yourself tested." I did, and I was—pregnant.

What I didn't know was someone had made an anonymous call to social services about the stuff going on at home. They sent a social worker to school to talk to me. I didn't want to tell anybody. I didn't want to uproot the whole family.

At the same time, someone from social services went to my house. They arrested my stepfather that very day.

I leave school, take the bus home, and walk into this.

My half-sister starts screaming, "*I hate you.*"

Andrew, my stepbrother, says, "Why did you say it was Dad?" This is his son. He can't believe it.

When my mom gets home from work, she starts screaming, too, "You're a liar! A liar!"

I felt terrible. I cried and cried.

At school, everybody stared at me. I knew they were saying I was disgusting. I didn't care. My close friends accepted me. I just kept going to school until a week before the baby was due.

The doctor said my amniotic fluid was very low. The baby didn't want to come out. They wanted to induce labor—make it start. They would give me medication to bring on contractions. Be at the hospital at 6:00 A.M., and I could bring my mother along.

At three in the afternoon, they took me off the medication. At four o'clock, my water broke. I said to my mother, "I feel like I have to go to the bathroom." I was in such pain.

I was a little more comfortable sitting on the port-o-potty. But then, all of a sudden, there was the baby's head. They shoved me into the delivery room and told the doctor. He came in at a dead run, and ten minutes later my baby was born. She had a full head of red hair and I named her Rusty Anne.

After I was home from the hospital for two weeks, my mom said, "I can't take this anymore. I want social services to put you in a foster home."

WHAT!?

It was like she kept me at home while I was pregnant. After Rusty was born, I could just go on my own.

A woman, a case worker, came from social services. She said, "We have a nice home for you with a nice foster-care family. I want you to take a look at it."

It was a young couple. They were only twenty-two and twenty-three themselves. They had three little kids. The state would pay them $300 a month each for Rusty and me, a total of $600.

That night, I packed all my stuff by myself. Next I packed what little I had for Rusty. In the morning we left to move in with that couple.

Within weeks, they were using me like a slave. Wash

dishes, cook, scrub the showers, wax the floor, clean the windows. On weekends, they had an even bigger list of things to do. Everything had to be spotless.

Rusty would cry. I'd let her go. The husband would yell, "Pick her up." But I thought picking up a baby every time teaches a bad lesson. And I wanted to raise her the way I thought best.

Three months after I had Rusty, I went back to school. I was in bad shape, tired and feeling guilty. I thought I should stay home with her, but how could I do that and get an education? I wanted to *excel*!

I'd come home with schoolwork, then stay up half the night 'cause Rusty was colicky. By then she was crying all the time. "Pick her up," the husband would holler.

My case worker stopped by to see how I was doing. She told me my stepfather had moved back in with my mom. Charges were brought against him, but he only got probation. "Don't worry," she said. "Things will be okay."

"What do I tell Rusty when she asks about her daddy?" I'd think to myself.

I was thirteen when I got pregnant. I was fourteen when I had Rusty. I was fifteen now and I wanted to have my own home. To learn how, I took some classes in Independent Living Skills.

"We'll find you a different foster family, instead," the case worker said.

And they did. The problem was the husband had been in Vietnam. He had flashbacks. He'd cry out in pain, like someone was kicking him. His wife was religious. She wanted him to go to this place where they get the Lord back into you.

Meanwhile, I felt like I never slept. I was always doing for Rusty, going to school, or studying. I never went out with friends. I had responsibility.

The only person I talked to during this whole time was Rusty. I'd sit there and cry.

"I'm trying to make all these people happy," I told her.

	WHAT'S FOSTER CARE?[1]
◯	Officials take children from their parents, usually because of neglect or abuse, and put them in private homes, group homes, or residential treatment centers. Foster care is supposed to be a temporary solution until the children are returned to their families or put up for adoption. However, many stay in the foster care system for years.

"I have to do well in school. It's our best hope for the future...."

She listened to me. She cried with me. It was like she understood me. When I stopped crying, she stopped crying. When I brought home my report card and was on the honor roll, we smiled together.

My foster mother thought I needed to get out a little. "Why not a part-time job?" she said. "Taco Bell needs help." I started working about five hours a night, four nights a week and weekends. At times I was working thirty to thirty-five hours a week. I loved it, but it was killing me.

Rusty went from day care to a nighttime babysitter. My foster mother said, "She's a disaster. Every time you leave the house, she screams her bloody head off."

She was two by now. She wouldn't sleep at night. When I was home, she followed me around like a lost puppy. I was irritable. She was irritable. My case worker was bugging me about parenting classes. I was getting, like, I can't handle this anymore.

On my sixteenth birthday, I bought myself a car.

I came home from work and my foster mother told me she had to spank Rusty to get her to bed. I looked at her and saw bruises. Bruises. I was upset.

My case worker and my foster mother said cut back on my work hours.

"Okay," I told them, even though I needed money for Rusty's diapers and clothes, and now car payments. I would try to get my life together, so Rusty wasn't a mess and the foster home could become a family again.

That worked for a week. I had to have my work. My work was my sanity. I was learning management, something good for my future.

I went to social services. "Look," I said, "I want to put Rusty in foster care by herself. I think it will be better for her. I'll catch my breath. I'll go live with my girlfriend and her mother."

It was a hot day. I dressed Rusty in a white jumper with a sailboat on it. I put her in the car and took her to another foster family. The new foster father came over to the car, opened the door, and unhooked the car seat. He took her away. No hug. No kiss. No good-bye. No nothing.

Rusty, my little two-year-old, turned back and looked at me, like, "What's going on?" I drove to my girlfriend's looking through my tears, flooded in the face with reality.

"My boyfriend was jailed for child abuse."

JUDY, 17 YEARS OLD

On New Year's Eve, I was with this guy, Eddie. I met him at the bowling alley the month before. He was visiting a friend in town. I thought he was nice. He laughed all the time.

I was curious about sex. It was one of those things. I just wanted to do it. An hour later, I went home.

When I missed a second period, I knew something was up. First, I thought, "Ohmigod, this can't happen." Then I decided, if I'm pregnant, I'm pregnant. I can't give it back.

I told Eddie, and he said he'd buy me a pregnancy test. He never got around to it. Then I told my sister, and added, "You have a big mouth. I want to keep it secret from Mom for a while."

Later that day, me and my sister were in the bathroom trying to curl our hair. We got in a fight. She got so mad she went running to Mom, "Judy's pregnant."

Mom screamed upstairs, "*You're what*?!" Well, she just threw a hissy fit. "How'd this happen?" she wanted to know.

"How do you think?" I said.

I felt abortion is cruel. I was going to have this baby.

Mom was kind to me once she got over the shock. She rented me a little apartment to live in and I went on welfare.

Pretty soon, though, Eddie and I got in this big fight. He broke up with me. He just didn't bother to let me know.

See, there was this girl, Donna. Her boyfriend kept beating on her. Eddie went to beat the beep out of him. After that, the two of them, Eddie and Donna, got together.

When I found out about all this, I told him, "I don't know what the hell you're doing. All I know is you were going with me. Now you're going on with someone else. No one does that to me."

Eddie said, "Well, if we're broke up, now I can go with Donna."

I was five months pregnant. Morning sickness sucked. Once that was over, it was cool. When you're pregnant, people are nice to you. No one gets on your case.

I started dating again. And guys *loved* that I was pregnant. They wanted to see how it felt to go out with a pregnant girl!

Then I got a call from a social worker. Because I was on welfare, they wanted to know about the baby's father. They had to have it for paternity papers. The only thing I knew was his name. I told them the truth, "I heard he left the state."

By then, I had started dating Max. None of my friends liked him. He hadn't gone past eleventh grade. I dropped out of school, too.

I wanted to spend time with my sister. Max wouldn't let me. But he was there for me. He showed up. He came to the hospital.

People tell you, "Oh, giving birth is great. The pain's not that hard." They lie. Childbirth hurts. Finally, I had a baby girl, Shannon.

For about a month, I stayed with Max at his home. It was his mother, me, him, and the baby. Then we moved three different times. Mainly, we stayed with friends for a while.

Max had a job at a pizzeria. I made him help with the baby, too. He'd get up in the morning, give it a bath, feed and change it. That's when I'd get up.

He started complaining, "That's your job."

"I get up in the middle of the night. You try that once in a while," I told him.

One morning, all I know was Max was changing the baby like usual. He picked her up by the arm and went to stick his other hand underneath her butt. By the time he started to do that, the baby wiggled around and started screaming.

She kept screaming, really long. Shannon has a high-pitched scream. Usually, you pick her up, hold her, and she stops crying. This time she didn't. And she wouldn't move her arm. I knew something was wrong.

The doctor took a look and said her arm was broke. Well, then, out of nowhere, protective services got involved. They came to the hospital and asked, "What happened?" We told them the story.

I can't remember exactly what they said, something about neglect and abuse. "We've got to take your baby away, put her in a foster home," they said.

I started crying, "Give me my baby back." She was just three months old. I thought I was being a good mother.

We went home. It was hard seeing the crib there and everything. I couldn't get to sleep that night. The doctor gave me "dry pills" to take, so the milk in my boobs wouldn't hurt that much.

There was a hearing. I had to go into the court and talk to a judge. He asked me a bunch of stuff, like, explain what happened. He said, "You're going to have to go to parenting class...."

Then the judge said I had to see Shannon one hour twice a week and all this mumbo-jumbo talk that they do. Next Max had to go to court. It was scary.

<table>
<tr><td></td><td colspan="2">**EFFECTS FROM CHILDHOOD ABUSE**[2]</td></tr>
<tr><td>○</td><td colspan="2">In their preschool years, abused or severely neglected children are more likely to get angry, refuse to follow instructions, and lack enthusiasm. By the time they enter school, they lack self-control and are easily distracted. They have a higher risk of depression, suicide, and drug problems. When they are teenagers, abused children are more likely to be arrested and more often for a violent crime.</td></tr>
</table>

Judges always put different words in there. You say it and they say it and it comes out different. The judge said, "How could you do that to a baby? You'll spend thirty days in jail—child abuse, second degree."

I've seen babies fall off of changing tables all the time. They break a leg or something. I don't see protective services jumping on them. It's just like with certain people they do.

I think they came after me 'cause I'm a teenager. It isn't any of their business. I should be able to raise my kid the way I want. I hate it when people get involved in your problems when you don't want them to.

When Max was in jail, I wrote him a letter. I said it wasn't working out between us. He wrote me, saying, "Well, can we be friends?"

Now he's out and he won't even talk to me. He's got a loose screw somewhere. I wanted him to say, "I'm sorry for what happened to the baby."

Then I could say, "Yeah, right." But I didn't hear any apologies.

Sometimes I think about what to tell Shannon about her dad. I'll say, "Yeah, you do have a dad. Somewhere around these United States. Someday you might see him. It just didn't work out between us."

To me, a guy's a guy. You've got to expect that from them. I won't throw my anger up to my kid.

But it's weird now. I live by myself in a downstairs apartment. I don't even have cable TV. I'm lonely. For money, since I went back to school, I'm on GA—general assistance. That's about the same as ADC [Aid to Dependent Children].

I go back to court September 19th. I should be able to get my baby back within that month. Shannon's a year old now.

I pick her up from the foster home. She's walking all over the place. I got a stroller so I can take her over to my friends to show her off.

I'd like to have a boyfriend. I like being with someone. It's fun—share the laughter, share the joy. What's important, too, is I want to be a good parent. That's all I've got to say.

"My son and I are in foster care."

MICHELLE, 16 YEARS OLD

Before I got pregnant, my life was sad. My dad was always sure I was sleeping with all these guys. He called me a whore. He tried to control my life. I couldn't even walk out of the house without him watching me.

Across the street from where we lived was a playground. Back then, I loved to swing. When I would swing, it was peaceful. Swinging took everything away. My dad realized that and said, "The farthest you go is the porch."

I was thirteen when I got pregnant. His name was Sam. He was twenty-seven, a friend of my dad's. We were running an errand together for him. Sam said, "Let's go up to my house for a minute."

We had sex. I didn't want to, but I was, like, "Oh, well, I guess I *am* a whore."

The next month I was spotting. I thought that was my period. I didn't know anything. I didn't actually comprehend what was happening until one morning I woke up and got sick.

A few minutes later, I was eating cereal. My mom said, "You're eating right after you threw up? Are you pregnant?" It was Saturday and my dad was there.

I was scared. He'd beat me before, lots of times. He beat my mom, too. That morning he took me into the basement and started hitting me with a board. He beat me until it broke. Then he got another board and beat me until I told him what happened.

He didn't believe me.

At school, I told my one friend, "I can't handle this anymore...."

She said, "You have to tell the counselor."

I finally agreed to tell her the truth. The counselor said, "I have to report it. Go to your classes and I'll send someone for you later." They took me out of my sixth-hour social studies.

An investigator came from the CPS, the Child Protective Services. They called in my mom and dad. They came to the office and turned on the tears. My dad said, "I don't know why she would say I ever beat her."

My mom was upset that I was pregnant. "Maybe that's why she's lying," she said.

The two of them told me to have an abortion; I was too young to have a baby. My mom said, "I had an abortion when I was thirteen, too."

"I'm not going to have an abortion," I told them. What nobody knew was that in a way, I was happy. If I had a baby, I had someone to live for. And this would be somebody who loved me.

The CPS gave me a physical. They said I was sixteen weeks pregnant. I couldn't go home. My dad was a danger to me. The CPS put me in a foster home. I was only supposed to be there for three days, but the family liked me.

That foster mom and dad went with me for the birth.

For me, the pain started all of a sudden. It felt like real bad period cramps. That's the basic area that I had them in. Of course, some girls have back labor pains, too.

The pain keeps getting worse and worse. And I can take pain.

I'd get a contraction. It would be a high one, and even before it went down, another would start coming. I was having two at a time every three minutes. The contractions broke my water. Your stomach tightens up, like it's a water balloon, and then it pops.

At first, the doctors didn't think I'd be able to carry the baby full term. They said I was too depressed. But I had a normal pregnancy and the baby came out healthy. I had a handsome, light-skinned boy, just like me. He had real good hair, too. I named him Kyle Matthew.

Kyle's two now, and we've been in about five foster families. I left that first place for these reasons. We had conflicts about how to raise a child. Also, they're white and I'm black—well, half black.

My mom's black and my dad's white. But I feel more comfortable around black families. I want Kyle to know he has many races in him. Sam, his dad, is a mix, too—part black, part white, part Navajo Indian.

After that first foster family, I went to one for about a week. The woman there was weird. We had to go to bed at eight o'clock. We couldn't go anywhere.

Then I went to a foster home where there were already five foster kids. There were three of us in the bedroom. I was hoping I could have my own room with my baby. Right from the start, the other girl was trouble.

She called me a bitch. I was ready to fight. I had to leave, though, for a doctor's appointment. When I came back, she had stolen my clothes, tapes, razor, and pressing comb. The foster mother said, "She's done that before."

I was, like, "Well?"

Two weeks later, I was out of there.

Finally, I found a place for me and Kyle where we stayed a while. I tried to get a routine. Every morning, before I took Kyle to school, I fed him some baby food. The foster mother came in one day and said, "You should cook him some bacon and eggs."

I got up at five in the morning to get ready for school. I didn't have time to cook him anything to eat. Just getting all our stuff ready took that long.

"Cook him breakfast or you're not going to the football game tonight," she said.

"What are you talking about?!"

"Your son must be your first priority."

I didn't understand what was happening. I wanted to go to this game. "Why are you doing this?" I said. "I feed him baby food every morning and you never said anything before."

I was her first foster child and we were not getting along. They sent me back to the home where the girl stole from me.

Kyle still wasn't sleeping through the night. The other foster kids hassled me about that. And the foster mother kept sending me mixed messages.

First she'd say, "You need to live out your teenage life. Give him up for adoption." Next she'd say, "You need to go be with the baby's father."

I called the social worker and said, "I'll sleep on a couch somewhere. Just get me out of here."

I hate being moved around. Every family has their own way of life. I feel like I'm intruding. I want to get a two-bedroom apartment. I want to raise Kyle right.

He's my sunshine. I love to watch him grow up. He could say "Mama" since about five or six months. He cut his first tooth when he was eight months. I helped him take his first steps at nine months. One day he just started counting. Oh, my word, I was so excited!

I admire myself. I feel I have gone through a lot of stuff in my life. But I don't have time to sit around wishing and crying.

I made a decision. I am not going to end up like my mom. I keep doing for my son even when I'm so tired it hurts. A mother has to take care of her children. They can't do it alone.

I *have* to go to school. I have to graduate. I have to get a good job. Because I have to take care of my son. Kyle inspires me.

"Four of my kids are in foster care."

ORALIA, 20 YEARS OLD

I used to read romance novels. The girl winds up getting pregnant. The guy leaves, goes away on a ship. Two years later, he's back. Everything is merry. He's delighted they have a child

Malarkey. That only happens in books, not real life.

I know. I was molested starting at the age of five. I was on my own at fifteen. Now I'm twenty and have FIVE children. Four of them are in foster care.

Let me tell you, today I'm realistic about life, what's surrounding me. Being a teenage parent is *no... piece...of...cake.* If you decide to become a teen mother, you hang up being a teenager.

The first time I was pregnant, I was fifteen. I was scared and happy. I think all women go through that stage where they wonder, Can I conceive? Can I have a child?

Unfortunately, though, my baby's father was a drug pusher. I was having aggravation and problems. I didn't want to eat. I wasn't taking care of myself. And then I fell.

A week later, I miscarried at home. It was painful. There was a lot of blood and blood clots. The fetus came out real dry. It just plopped in the toilet. I didn't know what was happening. Afterwards, I went to the hospital and was scraped inside my uterus.

I started thinking, "Maybe it's for the best. When the father isn't on the drugs, he's missing drugs."

I was just lingering around then. I thought about going back to school. I had quit because I kept throwing up.

If you want to consider it work—working numbers—that's what I did for money. Basically, I depended on the guys. When I had a boyfriend, it was, "You got money. I'm with you. You give me money."

Within a couple months, I was pregnant again. This time the father was my boyfriend, Victor. I was staying at my mom's then, on an open-and-close sofa bed. I told her, "I don't know what's come over me. Victor's an incompetent fool!"

"Give him a chance," she said. "He seems like a nice guy. He doesn't get high. So what, he can't keep a job. That's because he doesn't have a vocation."

"He's doing nothing with his life, Mom."

But she kept persisting. Anyway, I was five months pregnant and getting severe back pains. I was like, ow, oww, *oowww*. I was going into premature labor.

I went to the hospital and they did a sonogram. *Twins!* The doctor told me that to keep the pregnancy going, I had to take medication and stay in bed. Imagine. Here I am sixteen. I don't want to be cooped up in the apartment. My mother said, "Stay in bed."

I wanted to have natural childbirth, to see my kids come to this earth. But I couldn't. One of the babies had his feet first. They gave me a shot, what's called an epidural. That allows you to stay up while you're giving birth.

Then I had a Caesarian, a C-section. I laid there while they cut me open. I felt the pressure of them pulling out the babies. I heard a sigh. I heard a wild, crazy cry. I saw one baby, two babies. After that, I passed out.

Sometimes I feel that's the last time I really slept.

I go home to my mother's with two kids. And in some ways, I'm a kid. Who the *hell* knows about postpartum depression? Back then, I'm not even aware that it exists.

I constantly call this friend who works at a child development program. I tell her, "One baby's got to be changed and then the other one's got to be changed! I know a lot of girls say, 'I could fuckin' kill 'em,' but I can't take it out on my babies. I brought this on myself. I had no business having any children!"

My friend says, "Take a deep breath. Calm down. You're by yourself. You have *two* babies, not just one. You're going through some hormone changes...."

I don't know how long that depression lasted, because six months later, I got pregnant again. It was Victor, again, with his sad, droopy eyes. I knew it could happen. I was so blue, it was FUCK everything.

I never thought about getting control of my feelings. I never thought, What is it I really want? Think of the pros and the cons of having a child. If I do this, this is going to happen.

I just said, "Shit, I'm gonna have a baby," and I had a baby.

There I was with three kids. I tried to make the best of it. I was still living at my mother's. I had an alcoholic brother and a drug addict brother living there, too. The addict was leaving me without food for my children. Stealing my Pampers diapers to sell them to get money for drugs. I left.

I went to what's called in New York City the Emergency Assistance Unit. They placed me and my babies in a hotel, and from there to another hotel. I stayed there for three months until they got me my own apartment.

Victor came in and out. It was more sexual than any kind of real relationship.

He had minimum wage jobs. They would jerk him. He'd quit. I ran numbers or dealt drugs. That's the only thing I knew.

I insisted that Victor do something with his life, like, "Why don't you try the military?" I finally got through to him. He enlisted and went away.

He came back for a Christmas visit and, being that he was my kids' father, I was still attracted to him. We had intercourse. Then this other guy was living with me. I was going to break up with him and go back with Victor, but he said, "No."

He forced himself on top of me. He was aggressive and rough. I couldn't believe it. Normally you don't hear that the person you live with forces you to have sex. It's called rape. I said, "You hurt me mentally and physically. Leave."

So he did. That's when I realized I was pregnant. Only three weeks, but believe me, with my experience, I knew. The problem was, I didn't know who was the father. I did know I wasn't ready for another child.

Victor was out of the picture. The other one was out. I was alone and depressed. My next-door neighbor said, "Sniffing [cocaine] here and there will help you get through."

I started dating Rafael, a pusher...and I lied to him. By the time I told him I was pregnant, he thought it was his. Rafael started helping me out.

I didn't understand that I'm the kind who relies on someone or something to sustain me. With me and men, I'm an extremist. I do everything to please that person. I never work on loving myself.

I depend on a man's companionship to be happy. I depend on cigarettes to relieve me. I depend on my children to give me love.

All I understood back then was I was depressed.

When I did coke and then crack, it made me forget what was going on. I forgot the changes I was going through, the problems that were totaling up.

Rafael was arrested for assault and robbery. I was picked up, too, and kept in jail for three months. (My kids went to live with relatives.) After they examined me, saw I was pregnant, I asked, "What about an abortion?"

"Forget it," they said. "The waiting list is enormous."

The day I got out of jail, I got high. That's the only thing I could think to do. I was eighteen years old with nowhere to go. I did not think what I was doing to that child inside me. I was relieving myself from all the pain.

Crack, though, can induce labor, early labor. When I was seven months pregnant, I had a tiny girl in a taxi on the way to the hospital. She weighed one pound and fifteen ounces. She came out addicted to drugs.

For the next five or so months, she was in intensive care. Did I visit her? Not really. I was still getting high and had a guilty conscience.

My other kids got taken away from me and put in foster care. The Child Welfare Administration—CWA—did it because of the drugs. It was obvious I was using drugs when I had that child.

One night I was getting *high, high, high*. I said to myself, "I don't want this anymore. It's too depressing. I've got to get help."

I took the stem and broke it.

I went to a program, but I thought I could still hang out, drink liquor, and smoke weed. That would distract me from the cocaine.

Then I noticed some people smoking crack. I just went over and said, "Oh, give me a hit." I relapsed. I quit. I relapsed. I quit. I relapsed. I quit.

And I got pregnant. Number five.

"Get help," I said to myself "wherever you can find it. Get help from as many people as you can. Family. Friends. Associates. Strangers. Cry. Talk. Listen. Get help."

I found a program with a long name: the Chemically Abusing Problem Adolescence Program, CAPA. I've been clean now for thirteen months. I've learned so much about myself coming to this program.

I say to you, find a program. Don't wait until you lose your kids, lose your home, lose your dignity. Get help immediately.

What I know now that I wish I knew before is that with CWA, they don't just take your children. They try to help them. Like, with my two-year-old, the one born premature when I was on crack, she still doesn't walk. They helped her get physical therapy.

You could also go to CWA and say, "Here are my children. I'm giving them to you to put in foster care. I'm overwhelmed. I need a drug program. I need parenting classes. I need a psychiatric evaluation. Whatever."

Those people will help you and hold your kids in foster care until you're ready to have them back. It's better than if *they* snatch your kids and say, "We heard you have a drug problem. We heard you abuse your kids. We heard blah blah blah...." It's much harder to get them back when CWA takes them from you.

I'm living with my mother again, along with my new little butterball baby, Ruben. He's six months old. I feel much better about myself.

There's nothing I can do to change what's happened. I wish you would believe me when I say a dedicated, devoted parent should be an adult. An adult where they enjoyed their youth and then said, "I'm ready to be a mother. I'm ready to be a father."

I wish I practiced birth control, of course. I wish I waited until my life was more established, until some of my dreams and my goals were fulfilled. I wish I waited until I had explored, experienced, and tasted what life had to offer me.

But I didn't. And that's my real story.

PART V

Adoption

Basically, there are two kinds of adoption: private and agency. With a private adoption, you go through an attorney. With an agency adoption, you go through a private agency—such as ours, Spence-Chapin—or a public one—such as a government agency, a county department of social services.

To find adoption agencies, look in the yellow pages of the telephone directory under "Adoption" or "Social Services." School counselors, women's health clinics, and teen parenting networks can help you, too.

Those of us at adoption agencies are not here to talk you into anything. We're not here to talk you out of anything. What we try to do is prepare you for the choices you need to make.

Most teenagers hope they're not pregnant. You hope your period is just irregular. That means a lot of our clients don't come to us until the sixth, seventh, eighth month of pregnancy.

You wait beyond the time you can have an abortion. Then you're faced with raising the baby yourself or placing the baby for adoption. And you're not sure how you feel about adoption. Some say you see it as being selfish, irresponsible, and abandoning the baby.

If you feel that way, I ask, "What does a good parent do?"

Usually I hear, "A good parent takes care of the baby. You make sure it gets fed, clothed, and loved—and that it's taught the things it needs to know."

I say to you, "Isn't that what you're doing? A good parent provides for a child. You're providing a loving, adoptive family."

You should not feel guilty if you don't feel ready to be a parent. It's okay to want to do the things that teenagers do.

The sooner you contact an adoption agency, the more we can help you. For example, we talk about decision-making. We answer your questions.

One question we hear a lot is: Do my parents have to know about the pregnancy and adoption? We *strongly* suggest that, especially if you live at home, you involve your parents.

Most teenagers think, "My parents will kill me. They'll kick me out of the house." Rarely does that happen. Sure, there's some anger, some shock. But we hear from most girls that the parents are supportive.

However, some of you grow up with abusive parents. Well, there's nothing in the law that says they have to know. In fact, this is one of the few situations where you, a minor, can sign a contract—the paper giving up the child. Legally, the child is yours.

Another question we hear is: Does *he* have to know? Many times it was not a serious relationship. Or it's over, and now you've found out you're pregnant. No matter who did the breaking up, you've got bad feelings.

We help you separate out *those* feelings and think about how this child is going to feel growing up when it says, "What did my daddy look like? What ethnic background am I? Can I inherit any medical condition from him?" For the baby's future, we need to get information about both parents.

Let's say the birth father doesn't want to get involved at all. We say to you, the birth mother, "Could you take this medical form and have him or his family fill it out leaving off the name?" In many states, though, you have to name him.

When you fill out the form, you should be open and up-front. If you're crack-addicted, let us know. If you have childhood diabetes in your family, let us know. If this baby is the result of incest, let us know.

We may have to say to you, we don't have any families that can accept the baby at this moment. But we'll work with you to find an organization or a family that will take this child.

If you come to us, we ask you what you want in an adoptive family. Maybe you say, "I want them to be Catholic. I want them to live in the suburbs and be under forty. I want them to be college graduates, artistic, athletic, and have a dog."

We then give you information about several families that meet your criteria. The material often includes how the couple met and why they were attracted. It gives a physical description, education, and jobs. You can talk to your boyfriend, your parents, your friends to help you decide which family sounds best.

In some cases, you might want to meet the potential adoptive parents. These meetings don't always go the way you expect, but they're all wonderful.

Mostly you get funny, charming, articulate adoptive couples who suddenly become zombies. They're so afraid they're going to say the wrong word or they've worn the wrong thing, they get anxious. But, then, so do you.

Some agencies and private lawyers feel that teenage birth mothers aren't mature enough to make the decision on which family is right for their baby. They don't want you to meet. Ask the agency or lawyer you're thinking of going through, "What's your policy on this?"

Pregnancy makes you feel fat, makes it difficult to sleep. It puts you out of parts of your life you don't want to miss. Often there's a lot of feelings of anger, frustration, sadness, and *why me?*

One day, though, a baby is born. You're dealing with your flesh and blood. It's a different set of feelings. This is one of the most crucial and difficult times for the birth mother.

In most *private* adoptions, through an attorney, the birth mother signs the papers in the hospital. The baby is discharged and goes immediately to the adoptive family.

With Spence-Chapin and many other *agency* adoptions, we give the birth mother a period of a few days, a few weeks, or even a few months where the baby is put in temporary child care.

You've just gone through childbirth. It can be difficult under the best circumstances. You're under medication. You're not feeling well. You have incredible highs and lows. We feel this is not always the right time to make such a serious choice. You need to distance yourself to make sure this is what you want.

The decision to place a child in adoption—or raise a child by yourself—is one you have to live with for the rest of your life. We want you to feel good about it. We want you to feel comfortable, pleased, and confident.

At this point, the vast majority of birth mothers change their minds. They keep the baby.

For those who do turn to adoption, state laws vary about the formal procedure for signing surrender papers. What you should know, though, is that once you sign the papers, there is no automatic, easy way to get the child back if you change your mind.

It's very difficult and painful and expensive for everyone. It would be much better if you take an extra couple of weeks to make sure your decision is solid.

I think some people feel, "Oh, I'll never get over this." The truth is, while you don't forget, you do learn to live with it. And with an agency's help, you learn to live with it in a much better way.

"It was too late for an abortion."

EMILY, 16 YEARS OLD

David's the first person I ever slept with. He's different than most guys. He isn't self-centered and always talking about himself. He isn't macho. He's just nice.

For months, I told myself a million reasons why there was no way I could be pregnant, especially since David used a condom. Finally, I knew I had to move on it. At the time, I was not going to tell my parents. I was set on getting an abortion.

I cut school and went to a women's health clinic. I'd never been to a gynecologist before. I was scared of the demonstrators. Once inside, I was shuffled around to different people. First, one lady filled out an application, another did a blood and urine test, another did the examination, and another talked to me.

The doctor said, "You're twenty-one weeks pregnant. How could you let this go so late?! We can't legally do this."

I was hysterical. In my mind, I wanted it to be over. I didn't want anybody to know. I had tried to make decisions by myself with David.

A counselor said, "If you still want to get it done, you could go to New York State. It's legal there up to twenty-four weeks. It's a hospital procedure, though. You have to be admitted and stay overnight."

The more she told me, the more freaked I got: Be prepared for demonstrators outside. It's not some comfy hospital room. You're in a room with a bunch of other women. What it is, more or less, is they give you a saline solution that forces you to miscarry .

I'd been a wreck about getting an abortion, borrowing the money from David's best friend, and now I was, like, forget it.

I told my parents. David told his. All of them were upset, but they were more worried about him and me. How could we go through all those months hurting ourselves without telling them?

I remember my dad came into my room and said, "We're going to figure everything out."

I'm so sorry. I never wanted to disappoint anyone," I told him.

David was scared to death to come into my house. He was afraid my parents would hate him. But they knew and loved him. They never gave either of us ultimatums. Finally, me, my mother, my father, and David sat down and talked about options.

"If you decide to keep the baby," my mom said, "you could still go to school. You could still go to college. We'll help you as much as we can with watching her. We'll support you financially as much as possible."

"Keeping it is not an option," I said. One or two friends had done that. It was just not the way I wanted my life or a baby's life to be. It was unfair. Then I felt selfish: all I could think about was myself.

Still, I wanted a future. The baby would be more like my sister than my child. My parents would wind up raising her. Everyone's life at home, my sister and brother's, would be affected, too.

My mom said her doctor, a g.y.n., got hundreds of letters from couples asking if he knew of women who are pregnant and don't want to keep it. Finding a home for my baby—a white baby—would be no problem, he told her.

I felt the baby move.

The doctor wrote a letter to school, saying I needed home tutoring. I was "fatigued." I didn't want to have to deal with telling my friends. I just couldn't.

My mom went to see the lawyer the doctor suggested. How does adoption work? she wanted to know. What were my rights?

In the beginning, I didn't want to meet with Wendy and Harlan, the couple the doctor and lawyer said wanted to adopt the baby. David did. He wanted to know what kind of people they were.

Then I changed my mind. I did want a meeting. The word came back, they didn't want to see us. Well, I got annoyed. I said, "I don't mean to sound like a bitch, but I'm giving them something they can never have. I don't think I'm asking that much."

They set up a meeting.

It was awkward at first. Nobody knew what to say. I told them, "Please, don't feel like you're being interrogated. If you answer the question right, you win. You're the people we've decided on. We just want to know what you're like."

After talking a while, you could tell they really *liked* as well as loved each other. They liked doing stuff together. And then they asked things about David and me.

They said they'd tell the child about meeting with us.

You know, David was wonderful during this whole thing. Everyone was so worried about me that none of our parents saw how much he was going through. He was always calming me down. And he was scared that, God forbid, something might happen to me. I tried to let him know how much I appreciated all his support.

The doctor said, "Whenever your contractions are five minutes apart for an hour, or your water breaks, go to the hospital."

I was in bed, staring at the ceiling, when the twinges started. I woke up my mom and said, "We should go!"

"Relax," she told me.

I called David and told his mom I was ready. My dad walked the dog. I started throwing up. My mom said, "Don't worry. There's no more pain than very bad cramps."

That's not true! I was in agony.

After the birth of a baby girl, I felt lousy. I'd had an episiotomy. I had stitches and stuff. I was exhausted.

The nurses on the floor knew about the adoption. They put me in a room at the end of the wing by myself. That way, I didn't have to deal with other women and their new babies.

The lawyer wanted me to sign some papers. He'd take the baby to the couple. I was nervous. I went down to the nursery with David to see her.

Later, when I asked, a nurse brought the baby to my room. I looked at her. I played with her. I didn't hold her. I thought that was best. I didn't want to get attached to her.

I started to get depressed. I could hear women with their babies, giggling and cooing. I remember crying, saying to David, "I don't know what I want to do."

"You need time to decide."

They all knew I was getting more depressed. It was agreed the baby would be put in boarding care for a month while I thought about my decision.

My mom said, "You may not want to keep her as far as how you'd have to adjust your life. But, if you're going to hurt every day because you miss her so much...."

The whole time I was pregnant, I was convinced it was a boy. Having a girl made the decision harder for me. What if I never had another girl? What if I couldn't have any more children?

Meanwhile, the lawyer kept reminding me these people were both making over $100,000 a year. They could financially care for her better than I could. That annoyed me.

It wasn't as if she'd starve if I raised her. I was envious of them for being *able* to have her. I wished I could have been married. I wished it was later in my life when I could have kept her.

In the end, I felt I had no choice but to give her up. In my heart, as much as I was depressed and sad, I always knew I was going to give her up. It would be for the best.

A month after I gave birth, I went in front of a judge to sign the surrender papers. She asked me if I understood everything. At that point, I was giving up my legal rights to the baby, but I did have thirty days to appeal it.

For the first thirty days when she was in boarding care, I could have changed my mind and taken her just like that. The judge said, "After you sign these papers, if, for some reason you change your mind, you will have to appeal it and go to court. The court will then decide who gets the baby."

She said again, if I signed this, that has to be final. I wasn't thinking, "Ohmigod, I'm signing her away." I just did it. I was anxious for us both to get on with our lives.

It's been six months now. It feels long ago. I think David and I try to forget about it most of the time. In daily life we go to school, go to work, things like that.

I get depressed now and then. And when I'm upset about other things, I start to think about her.

Yesterday I was watching a rerun of "The Days and Nights of Molly Dodd." In the episode I saw, Molly just found out she was pregnant. I cried. I cried for me and the baby who will never know me. Will she hate me?

BETH, ADOPTIVE MOTHER,

PRIVATE INDEPENDENT ADOPTION

Four years ago, my husband and I adopted a baby. We named him Lucas. Now we're trying to adopt another child.

Like most adoptive parents, first we went through such a nightmare trying to have a baby. I had miscarriages, ectopic pregnancies, and years of tests. Not being able to make a baby is heartbreaking.

Finally, we decided to try to adopt. Instead of going through an agency where you wait and wait for them to call you, we went to an attorney who specializes in independent adoptions. He told us what to do.

We take out personal ads in newspapers. They say: "Happily married, financially secure couple looking to adopt a newborn. Please call the following number. Let us help you."

We have a phone number just for those calls. When that phone rings, we're scared. We want this baby more than anything in the world. And we don't know who's calling. Are you for real?

You should understand something important. This method of adoption has become well-known. A lot of not-very-together people make a lot of phony calls. These kinds of calls are cruel.

Because of them, sometimes the person who calls—

maybe someone like you—is questioned a little too closely. Just remember, we only want to know the truth. It's so important that you're honest.

In this first phone call, we ask for a few details. What happened? Why are you giving the baby up? How's your health? Have you been to the doctor? Are you sure you want to do this? Describe yourself. Describe the birth father, if you can. Not all birth mothers are sure who the father is. That's okay, too.

I know you're probably nervous answering these questions. You think, "These successful adults are going to be sitting in judgment of me. And here I am pregnant!"

Neither of us on this end of the phone thinks you're stupid or horrible. We've all had a sex life. Maybe we didn't get pregnant by accident, but the reason might have been that we couldn't get pregnant at all.

Usually we hear from someone who's about four or five months pregnant. And yes, you're going through a rough time. Frankly, though, I respect you for trying to make the best decision for the future of the child. You're responsible and caring.

Callers ask me questions, too. I hear, "Will you tell the child that he's adopted?"

"Of course," I answer. Lucas is four and we have begun talking to him about it. We describe it to him in the most *loving* way. We say he didn't grow in my belly. He grew in someone else's. She loved him and couldn't take care of him.

As he gets older, we'll give him more details.

Some callers worry that we'll tell the baby that they didn't care. Or that they were bad people. No adoptive parent would ever do that. It's not good for the child.

One young woman asks a special question. She wants to see if I'm capable of loving a baby I didn't make.

She says, "Describe how you felt when they put your son in your arms."

ADOPTION REGISTRY[4]

Until recently, confidentiality was guaranteed to birth mothers who placed their children in adoption. Now some states are passing laws giving certain rights to those who are adopted. At present, twenty-two states have set up a registry system aimed at matching birth parents and their adult children if both of them contact the registry saying they want to meet.

"It was the most extraordinarily happy moment in my life," I answer.

After this first conversation, we give you our attorney's number to call. That's where you should expect to really get grilled. The attorney asks about everything from your nationality to any drug use during pregnancy.

There's a long list of medical problems he checks off, including anything else we should know about your own family, and the birth father's family. Does the birth father know about this, and if so, how does he feel? Would he be willing to sign the appropriate forms?

Unless you're in the same city, this interview usually is not done in person. At some point, though, our attorney sends you to another attorney in your hometown to make sure everything is in order.

And certainly, before any money is given to you to help out, say, with medical expenses, basic living costs, and so on, you have to go to a doctor. You do this to confirm the pregnancy. You see, some people call and pretend they're pregnant just to get money.

You can call adoptive parents and talk to them and not be sure about adoption. You can talk to an attorney and not be sure. But once you commit to adoption, once you're heading down that road, you're involving other people. You have to come to terms with what you're doing.

In our own way, with our financial and emotional commitment, we're pregnant with you. We're expecting this baby, too. Last time we bought stuff for a nursery and kept it in my friend's garage. Up until we actually had the baby in our arms, we were terrified it was not going to happen, that the woman would change her mind.

This time, the young woman is due in six weeks. And between you and me, I don't know if she's going to give us the baby. While we're very sympathetic to her indecision and fears, we're terrified again. We feel vulnerable.

I start feeling depressed over not having been able to do this magical thing—have a child—myself. I pull myself up short with the following thought:

If God on high came down and said, "It was a big mistake. You *can* make your own children. In fact, you can make three of them. The only thing is, you have to give up Lucas. He can't be in your life."

I absolutely wouldn't do it.

No matter how heartbroken I am over not being able to make a child, there is nothing in the world, no promise of any kind that would make me want to give up this son. There's no difference between the way I love Lucas and the way birth parents love a child.

"The father was disappearing."

KRISTI, 18 YEARS OLD

Call me Kristi. That's the name I gave to the baby before the couple took her. Twenty years from now, I want to show her this book. I'd like her to know what happened.

When I missed my period the end of March, as much as I did think about it, I tried to fill my mind with other things. It was my junior year. You know that's crucial in high school. The SATs were coming up. Kevin and I both planned to go to college.

I was a cheerleader. I did gymnastics. Kevin played basketball, baseball, golf. And he was tall and good-looking. He was my first-ever serious boyfriend that I loved.

Right from the start, I told him I thought I was pregnant. He shunned it away, saying, "Well, maybe it's not true."

I'd go, "Yes it is, and I don't know what to do."

I knew that waiting wasn't going to help. But I didn't want to tell my parents. We were so close. I felt it would crush them. Instead, I told my aunt.

We looked at the calendar and tried to figure out how long it'd been. Then I asked her, would she take me to get an abortion? I didn't really want one. I thought, "If I have an abortion, when I die, I won't go to heaven to see my parents."

But Kevin and I didn't know how we could raise this child.

My aunt said, "You have to tell your parents."

That night, I told them. I wanted Kevin to be there with me, but he said he felt funny. And me, being so in love with him, I was *blind* to the way he was acting.

Anyway, my dad didn't say much. My mother kept saying, "Why didn't you come to me before?" She got in bed with me and we were up all night.

I was crying. She was crying. "I don't want you to be mad at me," I said. "I love you. I'm sorry."

Even though we're Catholic, my mother said, "Tomorrow we'll find out about an abortion."

Outside the health clinic, there're demonstrators. They yell at us: "*Murderers.*"

A lady sings "The Greatest Love of All," that song by Whitney Houston, "I believe that children are our future...." I break down.

I think to myself, "Hey, look, this is my life. You can protest. But I can be here and do what I want, too."

The counselor says, "You're about twenty-two weeks pregnant. We can't do an abortion that late in this state. There are a few places in Georgia...."

The reality hits me. I'm going to have a child. Everybody's going to know about it. I'm scared and upset. My mother says, "We're not going to risk an abortion."

As soon as I'm home, I call Kevin. He comes over and tells my father, "I love Kristi. I'll be with her through this whole thing." We all sit down to talk. The fewer people that know about it, the better, I think. Sure, if Kevin wants to tell his parents, he can.

He says, "No." They're strict. His mother wouldn't be able to handle it.

I think, "That's ridiculous. My mother has to go through it."

My mother made an appointment for me with her gynecologist. I'd never even had a g.y.n. exam.

We asked him about adoption. Not that I wouldn't have loved this child, but I wanted her to have a mother and a father—a *family*, like I did—and not a parent who was a teenage girl.

He suggested I go through an attorney. My mother had a friend who'd adopted a child through an agency. She said, "Families do so much to get a child."

We called a few agencies and had information sent to us. The one we chose would come here, to our home. I wouldn't have to go to the city to see them. By then, my parents were helping me make decisions. It was a load off my mind.

Right around then, Kevin started to act different. It was the first day of school. He picked me up. I thought I looked good. I asked him, "What do you think? Can you tell that I'm pregnant?"

He was, like, "Oh, yeah. No." He was the one who said he'd be with me. Now he was hanging out with a different crowd, the *in* crowd. He acted snotty toward me.

This was the last thing I needed. I cried every day. It was my senior year. I went to a couple of cheerleader practices, just to watch. I told everyone I had mono. The end of September, I quit going to school.

Carole, a lady from the adoption agency, came over and took information about me and Kevin. First, she asked about our family's health history. Once she got those questions out of the way, we talked about our situation and what we should do.

It was uncomfortable. I could tell there was tension between me and Kevin. He's not much of a talker. I am. But I wanted him to say... *anything*. Instead, he just agreed with me. He was not interested in being there.

That was the only time he met with Carole.

I had weekly visits with her. And we always talked about Kevin. He was disappearing and I didn't know what to do. Sometimes we talked on the phone, but he never asked how I was doing.

Say, he was freaked out. Well, there was help for him. Besides Carole, my father was willing to talk to him man-to-man. Once they were supposed to have breakfast and Kevin didn't show up. The same thing happened with my uncle. He waited an hour.

Carole asks me what kind of family I have in mind for the baby. I tell her, "Like mine." Irish background, Catholic, not that old. They don't need a lot of money, but I don't want them to be struggling.

My mother suggests we meet with one of the couples. They're nervous. I am, too. I'm talking and talking. I want them to get across to the child that it isn't that I don't love her.

"Will you send me pictures every six months?" I ask.

"Yes," says Megan, the adoptive mother. But then she keeps saying, "My child. My child."

That upsets me. I think, "No, it's not yours."

I was in the hospital all day. At 11:13 that night I gave birth. My mom was in the delivery room. She said, "It's a girl!" She was the cutest little thing I'd ever seen.

She weighed six pounds five ounces when she was born. So did I. And so did my mother and my grandmother. My doctor recommended not seeing the baby, not touching her, not holding her, nothing.

But then I thought, "I'd go through my whole life wondering, 'What did she look like? What did she feel like?'" I talked to her, hoping that she would understand.

Maybe for some people, it would sway their opinion. At this point in adoption, you can change your mind. For me, I loved being with her.

One day Kevin came to the hospital. I took the blanket off the baby and showed him how long her legs were, her tiny hands. He held her. He was afraid. He said she was too small.

My mother, father, Kevin, a social worker, and a notary—someone that stamps the paper—came the day I was released from the hospital. We had to sign the first paper about the baby. The second one, the more important one, I signed thirty days later.

Kevin was holding my hand, comforting me. We both were crying. But because he was missing school, he said he had to leave right after.

I didn't find out until I was back at school in January that he was going out with someone else since the fall. I wanted to tell his parents about the baby. I knew they would *kill* him.

It's a year later. I think, "When I get married, what will I tell my husband? My children?" I have to be honest. And I don't know how he or any child would react.

I have stretch marks. That's not pleasant. I think, "What about Kevin?!" He gets away free. When I ask him if he's going to tell his parents, tell a future wife, he goes, "I don't know."

And I can't go a day without thinking about the baby.

I have a dream. I hope that when she grows up, she wants to meet me. I walk into a room and see "me." I say, "I love you."

PART VI

Parents

"We'd better last forever."

I've *always* had a boyfriend. I don't like being alone. But back when I was fourteen, before I met Peter, boyfriends sometimes meant trouble. We partied, did drugs, cut school. One month I was in class for only a day.

My parents always compared me to my "perfect" older brother. I didn't care. I wanted to do what I wanted to do.

Then Peter and I started to get serious. He picked me up every day. We walked each other to classes. We went to lunch together. After school we'd go to work and meet right after.

At night we either ate supper at my house or his. Then we'd go into his downstairs bedroom. We'd watch TV and whatever else. Every time we came upstairs, his mom and dad said, "You're going to have a problem that you're not going to be able to deal with."

Every time Peter said, "Don't worry."

We'd been going together for about eight months when I got pregnant. Since I couldn't get the nerve to tell my mother, Peter followed her into the kitchen and said, "Susan's seven weeks pregnant."

She shook her head and said, "Stupid kids. You should know better." She came into the living room where I was and said, "There's going to be *no* abortion."

"Fine. I want to have my own baby, anyway," I said. Then I started to cry. "I feel bad because I hurt you again."

"Don't feel bad for me," she said. "Feel bad for yourself."

Next we went over to Peter's. His dad was sleeping in front of the TV. His mom was sewing up a shirt. "I'm going to tell you something and you're not going to like it," Peter said.

She knew right away. "I warned you guys...." She told me I had to stay in school. That was important. Then she gave both of us a hug, cried a little, and said I'd better go see the doctor.

After that, I went to my doctor's office about once every month. Near the end, I went every other week. At first he gave me lots of pamphlets to read—like, if you're smoking, your baby is, too. What the risks are when somebody young gets pregnant. Sometimes you can't go full term or there are complications during delivery.

My weight was a surprise. I didn't look real heavy or pregnant, but when I got on the scale it just jumped right up. I gained thirty-eight pounds.

Each appointment the nurse would take my heartbeat, blood pressure, and see if I had any questions. She explained what was going on in my body. What was happening with the fetus. She said a baby can hear you when it's seven months along.

Around the end of my pregnancy, the stretch marks came. They're just miserable. They're red and look like rips in your skin. You think you can use cocoa butter or a cream from K-Mart that says it gets rid of them. I've tried everything. Nothing works.

The baby was supposed to be born July fourteenth. It was a week late. I was laying there watching my TV game shows when the contractions started getting hard. I had tears in my eyes.

We all went to the hospital, and when we got there, they said, "Well, you're not going to go for a while."

"Don't tell me that," I said. But then all of a sudden, the contractions were right on top of each other. Contractions are weird. You can't describe them. You think you're going to be prepared for them. You think of the worst pain, and it's worse. It's *unbelievable*.

But as soon as you see that baby, you forget them.

Misty's five months old now. I never thought it would be this hard. Everything is rush, rush, rush. I don't have any time for myself. I get up the first time at four in the morning.

She wakes me up. And I love my sleep. Well, Misty wants to eat.

I go to the kitchen, make a bottle, feed her and while I'm burping her, she falls back asleep. A couple of hours later, it's time to get up again.

We shower together. She gurgles the whole time. It's so cute. Then I wash her hair, dress her, and put her in a chair while I get myself ready.

By then I have ten minutes to get us out the door. I make three bottles, get five diapers, some bibs—she's teething. And an extra outfit—sometimes the poop comes out of her Pampers.

I put everything in a diaper bag, run it to the car, and come back for her. I throw on her snowsuit and hat, pick her up with a big blanket around her face, and race her out to the car seat.

I bring her to school with me. There's day care. The pregnant girls and teen mothers help each other. We try to prepare the pregnant ones a little.

I tell them, "You have to do what's best for your baby and not for you. Sometimes when I'm at my wit's end, my mom will watch her for a half hour so I can just go for a ride. Maybe you can do something like that, too."

When you're a mother, you have to *plan* everything. Like, if you can find that babysitter, great. If not, you have to sit home. You start getting used to that.

What's really a surprise, though, is how expensive a

child is. I have WIC, a government program where you get free baby formula. When I was pregnant, they gave me stuff, too, milk, juice, and certain foods—cheese, cereal, eggs, and peanut butter.

Now I get thirty-one cans of formula a month. That was fine in the beginning, but now Misty drinks about forty-two cans. And where I live, they cost two dollars a piece.

Diapers—mediums—cost eleven dollars for forty-four. She goes through that many in about a week and a half. That means I spend about forty dollars a month just on diapers.

With clothes, one little outfit usually costs about ten bucks. And that's probably the cheapest outfit you can find. Of course, you need socks, and in the winter you need a one-piece T-shirt, because when they're in two-piece outfits, you lift them up and their shirt goes up. For three T-shirts, that's ten dollars.

At school there's a box full of coupons for diapers and stuff. Sometimes you can find one for two dollars off, which is a big help. I used to laugh at my mom when she worried about coupons.

We talk about budgets in our Life Skills class. My monthly budget for clothing, food, and housing is $2,900. That's the problem. I only make minimum wage, and so does Peter.

After school, I grab all the bottles, put everything in the diaper bag and bring Misty home from school. My mom watches her from two-thirty to seven o'clock when I work. I don't know how I'd do it without my mother.

Afterwards I come home, feed Misty her cereal, eat supper myself, and play with her. I talk to her in weird voices. She looks me right in the eye, curls her little hand around my finger. We connect.

By ten o'clock she's in bed. We share my room. I used to think it was big. Now it's filled with a changing table, my bed, her crib, my dresser, her dresser, and toys.

When I finally stop, that's when I think most about

TEEN BIRTHS UP

An eighteen-year-long decline in teenage birth rates has suddenly reversed, with the biggest increase among mothers fifteen to seventeen years old.[1] Ten thousand, five hundred and eighty-eight teens under fifteen gave birth, as did 478,353 age fifteen to nineteen.[2] (Three hundred ninety thousand and seven hundred had abortions, and an estimated 131,540 miscarried.)[3]

Peter. A month ago, he went down to Texas to try to find better work.

I'm not used to having just myself. I'm used to Peter always being around. Our friends say, "You guys are gonna last forever."

We'd better! I don't know how single mothers make it.

"That baby is my flesh and blood."

JORDAN, 19 YEARS OLD

Nowadays, lots of young teenagers, thirteen, fourteen years old, want to live in the fast lane. Instead of taking care of business, they want pleasure. They want to party. Well, partying leads to sex and sex can lead to pregnancy.

I know, my lady was fourteen when she had my daughter, Zoraida. I was sixteen. But I couldn't leave them. That baby is my flesh and blood.

I was scared at first. Zoraida was so small. She'd be laying there, and then she was hungry. But so was I.

When you become a father, you learn you have to put your own needs second. Without thinking, a kid's got to come first. It's mandatory.

Being a good father means you have to be patient.

I want Zoraida to always know, even if me and her mother were to have some changes, I'm here to watch her grow. My father wasn't around much when I was young. He still just comes and goes.

His relatives would tell on my mother. Her relatives would tell on my father. He'd go live at his sister's house. She would set him up with women, when she knew he was married to my mother.

Maybe it wasn't my father's fault. I blame him, though. He's supposed to be the man. He's supposed to know that he's got kids around the corner with nothing in their mouths to eat. When my mother would ask him to help with money and stuff, he'd start a fight.

This is what I watched growing up. Still, my mother raised me right. I never got in any trouble.

I get on my knees and pray every night. I try to stay around people doing positive things. I pick up the phone and call other young fathers. We keep in touch with one another, keep communicating.

Having a baby made me and my lady responsible. We learned that real life is *not* about sex. Anyone can lie down and make babies. Life and relationships are more than that. We learned that we've got to show our love and have goals that we're trying to get to.

We said, "We'll stick together and stick it out."

Six weeks ago, we learned another lesson. Sometimes in a relationship, right and wrong come at you at the same time. That doesn't mean you're going to fall down and crumble up. You learn to stay strong.

We lost our new, two-month-old son. He was a healthy baby, weighed eight pounds and ten ounces when he was born.

I was at work. I'm an engineer technician. My lady was at home. She woke up and went to check on the baby.

He wasn't breathing.

She gave him mouth-to-mouth to try to save him. Too late. It was a crib death.

We don't blame each other. We just try to be with each other. It's no one's fault. Doctors don't really know why it happens. I told my lady, "God wanted our little boy."

My whole family went to the funeral. I took Zoraida up to see her brother. She reached over and said, "See, see, see." She thought he was asleep. Zoraida's too young to understand. When she gets older, we'll tell her.

As far as my lady, she's going through a depression. She's strong but shy. If she lets out her emotions, she does it on her own.

I keep talking to other fathers. They're really there for me. I let out my pain when I get by myself. I cry.

HUGHLETT POWELL, M.S.W.,

COORDINATOR, SERVICES FOR YOUNG FATHERS;

JOHN GOMEZ, M.S.W., SENIOR SOCIAL WORKER,

YOUNG FATHERS PROGRAM, YWCA, NEW YORK CITY

Hughlett Powell

The teen fathers you hear about in the news are the hit-and-run victimizers. The inseminators. They get a young woman pregnant, then disappear.

Our program sees those of you who don't get in the news. We welcome young fathers who want to be involved with your children. You're trying to accept your role.

We know you have many of the same worries as the young woman. "How am I going to tell my parents? They want me to go to college. I can't even take care of myself. How can I take care of a child?"

The trouble is, while there are lots of programs for teen mothers, in many cities there's no place for the fathers to go. It's up to you to ask a school counselor, a social worker, the mother of your child—do they know? Are there programs for you?

John Gomez

Asking for help is *not* a sign of weakness. It means you want to accept responsibility. Still, we know it's harder for a young man than a woman to say, "I need help."

When you do come to our program, what I first hear is, "I want a job." It's not until you sit down in our young fathers' group, where others are sharing their lives and their difficulties, that you start talking, too.

When you're a father, you feel pressures: housing, education, and, of course, employment. You might feel pressure from your new family. Do they only want you around for your money, for child support? You might feel pressure from your parents. Should you feel ashamed, guilty? You might think you've made the biggest mistake of your life.

Well, you should know you have choices. You can get your life together.

Hughlett Powell

A lot of you do see your worth in terms of how much money you can produce. And your female partner may constantly remind you. You're the breadwinner. You think being a good, responsible father is about providing a child with GAP clothes.

That's not true. Fatherhood is not just about dollars and cents. It's about emotional support, too. Even if you're out of work and frustrated, you can give of yourself.

Some of you come from families where there's violence. You think, "I see my dad hit my mom. I'm going to do the same thing in my own relationships." You may also believe your child can be pushed around, that corporal punishment, beating your child, is the answer to discipline. You're wrong on both counts.

All of you say, "I want much more for my children. I don't want them to go through what I've gone through." For you and your child to reach for a better life, you have to work at believing in yourself. You have to work at building up your own self-esteem.

Find a parenting program. Find a caring adult with solid information. Reach out for help.

"He told his parents the baby wasn't his."

NICOLETTE, 16 YEARS OLD

I don't know a thing about being a mother. It's hard to believe that I am one. I'd always planned to go to college to be a lawyer. Now I am learning about law—paternity law.

I was going on fifteen when I first had sex. In the beginning, James, my boyfriend then and the baby's father, was a sweetheart. I saw him almost every night. Still, he wasn't the type to talk about feelings or to use birth control.

We did it when he wanted to. When he was done, that was it. He didn't care if I got anything out of it.

Then one night, James accused me of going out behind his back. He called me a bitch and smacked me across the face. I was shocked. Nobody'd ever hit me before. I tried to get out of the car.

He forced me back in and started screaming. I cried, "Take me home." After that, we broke up, got back together, and broke up again.

We'd been having sex off and on for five months before I started getting sick. I had bad headaches. My legs ached, too. I was like, "Please, God, if You're nice, don't let me be pregnant."

By the time I found out I was pregnant, James and I had dwindled to where we were hardly speaking. We'd see each other in the hall and he'd look away.

I called him up after school and said, "I have something important to tell you." I thought I should tell him face-to-face, but he wouldn't come over.

Finally, I just said, "I'm going to have a baby." The *minute* he heard that, he yelled, "Don't blame me."

"I've never been with anybody in my life but you."

He started being nasty, like he used to. "This is all your fault. Why didn't you do something about it? Are you trying to ruin my life?"

After screaming at me for a half hour, he got quiet and said, "What do you expect me to do about it?"

"You're graduating. I have two years left. I need help. I expect you to help me a little bit."

"It's not mine," he answered. We never talked about it again until after Pamela was born, five months later.

My family was disappointed, but they've stuck by me. With my dad, though, I'm *his* baby. He's protective of me. He wanted me to go through life as well as I could. He thought a baby would hold me back. I told him no to abortion and to adoption, too.

My mom and dad thought that James should take some responsibility. They went and talked to his parents. His parents said, "He's already told us it's not his."

My mom said, "Nicolette wouldn't lie to us about something like this."

They said, "Our son has gotten in trouble before. But he's our son. We've got to believe in him. When the time comes, we'll make him get blood tests to prove whether he's the father...."

The day I had Pamela, my mom called his house. James answered. When she told him, he said, "okay," and hung up.

A few days after that, I called and asked him if he'd come see her. He wouldn't. That's the last time I talked to him.

Pamela looks identical to him. He's got sandy hair. She's got sandy hair. I know all babies are born with blue

	BRAIN FOOD[6]
◯	During the first year of life, a child's brain grows to two-thirds its final size. If a baby doesn't get good, healthy food during that critical period, she or he will need intensive help to repair the damage.

eyes, but his are greeny-blue and hers have already turned like that. Her mouth is shaped like his. Her nose.

Now here's the problem. I went on social services, ADC, Aid for Families With Dependent Children. I'm not poor. My family is not poor. But babies cost a lot of money. I just need a little extra until I can get some child support from James.

In my state, if you're on ADC, you have to prove paternity. That's because the father is going to have to pay back all that money.

For example, I have a medical card. By law, he has to pay back at least 50 percent of my expenses—all my bills when I was pregnant. Right now they're over two thousand dollars.

He can admit he's the father and sign a form. But he's stubborn. So there are blood tests. To prove paternity, they take blood from me, Pamela, and James. But we can't get a blood test until the baby is six months old. If he's proven the father, he has to pay for the test, and that's four hundred dollars more.

Meanwhile, I'm required to go talk to an attorney. She asks very personal questions. Things about what James and I did. And she's cold. She makes me feel like I did something wrong.

She acts like because I need money, because I have a baby, I'm stupid. I don't want to be cut down for all this. I'm not the only teenager to have a baby. And people don't have the right to act rude and insulting. But they do.

I'm not sure about my future. I'm not sure I still want to be a lawyer. I would never give up Pamela right now. But in a way, I wish I didn't have her.

Your model for parenting comes from your home. Unless you've hung around with other families and seen something different, what you're going to do with your own children is repeat what happened to you.

A good way to get more information on how to raise children is to take a course at a local high school. You can also talk to other parents, check for help at local clinics, and read books on the topic.

It's up to you to evaluate that information when it comes to your own baby. You want to make the best decisions to meet your baby's needs. And this includes understanding child development—how children change as they get older.

Let's look at some examples. Making sure that your children are safe includes taking them for medical examinations and getting them inoculations.

It also includes things such as your knowing that babies can't see danger. Never assume that even a two- or three-year-old can be left alone.

The parent's job is to provide safe limits. When children are too little to understand a dangerous situation, remove them from it. Put them in a playpen or remove the dangerous object and replace it with a safe object.

When children are a bit older and they're doing something you don't want them to do, use a distraction. Focus their attention on something else.

	NON-STOP CRYING[7]
○	Colic is characterized by crying that can go on for more than three hours at a time. It affects about 20 percent of all babies, usually when they're one to four months old. Researchers now think cow antibodies cause this. They can be passed on in milk-based formulas. Or if nursing mothers eat dairy products such as milk and cheese, the antibodies can be passed on in the breast milk.

You can put them behind a gate across the door of a room. You don't want to put them behind a solid, shut door. Children feel frightened by that. The object is *not* to scare your kids, but to set reasonable limits.

By the time children are about two, if they do something you don't like, you can start using what we call "time out." Time out is putting children in a place where they can still see you, but they have to sit for a brief period of time. The older the child, the longer the time out. For a two-year-old, about a minute is plenty.

What you're trying to do is teach your children self-control and self-discipline. And you're trying to do this without hitting them. I'm for discipline, but real discipline doesn't involve hitting a child. Once you start hitting, they're going to expect to be hit.

Parenting *is* a tough job. It can be frustrating. People respond to that frustration in different ways. Most people say, "If I'm frustrated, I try to take time out from the situation until I can collect myself. I try to exercise. I try to do things for myself away from the house. I try to seek information on how to solve my parenting problems."

But some people say, "I just can't stand it any more. I don't want to assume the responsibility." They respond to that frustration by becoming withdrawn and depressed. When that happens, you neglect your children.

There are warning signs that you may be neglecting your children. Your children complain a lot about physical problems. They have accidents. They aren't sleeping well. They look sad and withdrawn.

Sometimes people who have had abusive parents try to do the opposite of the family patterns. Because you *don't* want to repeat the abuse, you become neglectful parents. You don't know what else to do. If others are telling you that something's wrong with your children, that's a big warning sign of neglect. Listen to them and get help.

Some people respond to that frustration with anger and aggression. And then you get physical abuse. You don't always know you're physically abusive to your children. You just think you're doing what you should do to discipline them. You say you beat them to teach them not to beat somebody else. You're trying to make them be good people.

Warning signs of physical abuse would be that you scream at your children. You shake them. You hit them. You leave them unattended when they are in danger. If you recognize these signs, you should get help.

With sexual abuse, you're dealing with something different. Sexual abuse is interacting with a child in a way that stimulates or arouses you or the child. It's *completely* inappropriate. It's usually an addictive behavior on the part of the person who's doing it. And it's repetitive. If you do it once, you're going to do it again.

People who are sexually abusive to children know they are.

If you are a survivor of sexual abuse, without exception, you ought to go and talk to somebody about that. The biggest set-up for somebody to become abusive is to have been abused and to have not resolved it. That goes for men and women.

Nobody is going to care about or love your children more than you. And your children, when they're babies, need you to be at their side at all times. Until they can do for themselves, you're their eyes and their ears and their hands. Your children become the best people they can be— with *your* guidance.

"I didn't want to deal with it."

JOHN, 17 YEARS OLD

I was sixteen when Brook had a baby and I became a father. I felt like I was less of a man if I wasn't involved. But at the same time, I *knew* I didn't want to deal with it.

I was still living at home. And for months, Brook kept snapping at me that I wasn't helping. One night I say, "Okay, I'll take the baby all day tomorrow."

Well, the baby wakes up with a ruptured eardrum and before I can ask, "What's that?" Brook is giving me orders.

"Take the baby to the doctor, but first stop off at day care to explain why he won't be there."

I walk into day care and they're checking all the kids for head lice. I say, "Not my kid."

They say, "Stay a few minutes. One of the helpers is late."

Right away, this little girl comes up to me and says, "My tummy hurts." The next thing I know, she's lying on the floor in a puddle of vomit. I go up to one of the leaders and say, "That little girl puked. And by the way, I don't clean. I'm putting a desk over it."

They decide I'm not much help, after all. I leave and drive to the doctor's office, twenty minutes away. We don't have an appointment, but they'll squeeze him in.

Then, since Brook says she has no food in the house, I have to go buy groceries for her and the baby. I stop off to get the medicine for the ruptured eardrum. The guy behind the counter says, "Do you have a dropper?" That's how you put the medicine in.

I have no money for a dropper, and I don't know if Brook owns one. I get back in the car, the baby's screaming. I haven't changed his diaper since eight that morning and now it's afternoon. I won't go near it by now. Brook can change him.

I drive another twenty minutes to her place. I unload the groceries. Brook starts her usual snapping about diapers and medicine and dinner and put the baby to bed. I just about curl up. I shut down, stop talking.

She wants to know why I'm quiet as a cat. Why won't I help more with my son? What a dumb question. I'm gone.

RICK MULLEN,

GROUP CARE DIRECTOR,

FLORENCE CRITTENTON SERVICES,

SAN FRANCISCO

Across the country, there are about thirty organizations called Florence Crittenton Services. Each is independent. Each offers different services.

Here in San Francisco, we're a group home for pregnant teenagers eighteen or younger, as well as for teenage mothers and their children under the age of three. You can find out if there's a Florence Crittenton or similar type of residential home near you by asking a school counselor, a Planned Parenthood worker, a drug counselor, or a social services worker.

We're here to offer you opportunity, support, and help. We help you through your regular schooling, as well as provide information about prenatal care, nutrition, budgeting, and career development.

We're not a boarding house. You don't come and go as you please. There's also no drinking, no drugs, and no fighting. Health care is mandatory for you and your baby. You have to clean your room every day, attend a variety of group meetings, and live with the curfews. If you're late, there are no excuses.

There are consequences for your actions.

Many of you say you want to give your child the kind of mothering you never had. At the same time, you can't think having a baby is like getting a puppy—and it's always going to be a puppy.

MEASLES ALERT[8]

Measles cases are increasing and some are resulting in hospital stays and even death. When to vaccinate a baby for measles depends on whether there is an outbreak in your area. Check with a medical person. Normally, children should be vaccinated at fifteen months of age and again before they enter school.

Babies quickly turn into older children. With that comes a whole new set of responsibilities. Remember, you're the main person responsible for your children until they're grown. That's a heavy burden for anyone, especially a teenager.

Sometimes all I hear are pessimistic views about young parents. I want to say that it *can* work. I don't want to encourage you to have children. You give up so much. Still, I wouldn't want you to think that because you have a child your life is ruined.

I admire the girls who come here. Many come from difficult circumstances to begin with. They're very determined and work very hard. And they do it. You can, too.

"I'm there for my kids."

ANTHONY, 22 YEARS OLD

Oh, man, am I a father! There are three different mothers, three different kids, and one me. But I deal with it.

Along the way I've learned some stuff that, maybe, can help you, too. Let's deal first with when girls are pregnant. Some of them feel they're carrying all the burden. They get into *moods*. You're always hearing, "I'm fat. I'm ugly. I'm this. I'm that."

The pressure gets so much it's, like, pushing you away. That's when a lot of you begin to be sorry. You want to just lay the girls, make them pregnant, and run out the door. I say, "Be a *man*. Stick it out." You've got to handle the frustration of their taking out their feelings on you.

Tell them, "I'm there for you, and that child, too." At times, though, it's never enough. They treat you like a crumb inside a barrel of apples.

I've been there to see one of my babies born in the house. We couldn't make it to the hospital. The paramedic happened to be a reverend, too. He blessed my baby boy right there in the bedroom.

I've seen my two other babies, two girls, born in the hospitals. Whatever way it happens, I'm telling you, it is a shocker.

With one, the mother barely got through the emergency room doors and the baby came out. But with the very first one, I felt like the mother, Lisa, and I went through the whole thing—together.

I went to the wash-up outside the delivery room. I put on the blue surgical suit just like the doctors. They said she was going to have a C-section, a Caesarian section. I could go behind the glass and see all they were doing—blood and everything.

They had her stretched out with her arms locked to the sides of the operating table. They had these machines and monitors on Lisa. I watched them open her up. I saw the birth. I saw this funny-looking, snake-like thing—the umbilical cord. I saw the afterbirth.

When you see the baby, you can see right through, see the veins. I wondered, "How does the baby survive all that?" I got weak in the stomach. I fainted.

When I came to, I was lying in the bed next to Lisa in the recovery room. She'd gone through the operation, was cut open, sewed up, and wheeled back out.

At fifteen, I was a first-time father of a baby girl. Me and Lisa named her Dorian. I was so excited, I just about overheated. Everything, I figured, would be roses.

Another thing I learned is, good or bad, when you're a parent and it comes to your children, you've got to deal with it. Even if you're a perfect parent, kids get sick and hurt: asthma attacks, fevers, cuts, allergies, sore throats.

Once one of my kids was sick and we didn't know what was wrong. The mother, Kelly, said, "Maybe he has a cold or something. He's been in the house for two days."

We talked it over, and then we had to decide what to do. Finally I said, "He's going to the hospital."

So I'm coming in the hospital door and I'm in my T-shirt with my jacket wrapped around him. I walk straight into the emergency room. I don't even register. They start hassling me about documents for the baby. I keep saying, "But I'm his father. The mother is at her mother's house in Brooklyn with the papers."

The doctors are looking at me, looking at the baby. I hear one say something about child abuse. They want to call the police and I'm just trying to help my kid.

See, I didn't know until later that the baby had a 105.9 degree temperature—pneumonia and two ear infections. At the time, I didn't know it was such an emergency.

My parents are still married—for twenty-seven years. I'm not doing that well. And sometimes I think it comes down to interference.

Maybe Lisa would have been my only girlfriend or wife if I'd put my foot down and said, "Listen. The Joneses can be the Joneses. I'm not them. We can afford this. We can't afford that. Let's just be ourselves."

But Lisa's into her mother and her sisters. She was raised without her father being in the house. And because he was not there every day to talk to, to relate to, she tends to shy away from men.

We started arguing. My parents let me run my life, but they do give advice. My parents say, "In any relationship, no matter how extreme the problem is, give yourself time. Put it aside. Go back to it. Talk about it. Work on it."

All I heard from Lisa was, a man's supposed to do this. A man's supposed to do that. I was living at home, working for my father. I was still in school. I was seeing her and Dorian every day.

I felt I was accomplishing. I also felt I was being used. And any time a male feels that way, he's going to back up. "Enough is enough," I said to myself.

But then, I had to figure out how to keep seeing my

baby, Dorian, when me and Lisa were over. I knew it wasn't the materialistic things you give your children. It's the quality time you spend with them.

How could I talk to my child, play with my child, share things with her that I'd like her to know? Lisa told me she had other plans. She wanted to take my daughter and go on about her business. I felt terrible. I wanted to be there for Dorian.

I said, "Okay, you want to be in your world. I want to be in my world. But Dorian has still got to be in the middle."

After Lisa, I got involved with Kelly. She already had one son before she had ours. I told her, "I'm with you now. You've got my kid. I'll try to take care of the whole thing."

I felt good knowing that I could go out every day, work, and put food on the table. I didn't have to turn to my mother, my father. It was all me. I was doing things for my son.

With him and my daughter, I started learning more about kids' tricks. Kids like to play Mommy against Daddy and Daddy against Mommy. Meanwhile, Mommy and Daddy are standing there, looking at each other, saying, "Why did you do that? Why didn't you tell me first?"

What I try to do is this. Say Dorian tells me, "Daddy, I want to go to the movies."

I ask her, "What does your mother say about that?"

"Oh, Mommy says it's okay," she says.

Then I tell her, "Sweetheart, I'm not saying no, I'm saying maybe. First let me double-check with your mother. If she says all right, we'll go."

What you learn is kids lie. Her mother had already told Dorian "no way" to the movies. If I didn't check first, if I just went and got the tickets, Lisa and I would have been in another fight.

My advice is you and the children's mother should talk to each other before taking any action. I don't care if it's a single parent or both parents under the same roof, you have to keep communicating. And that link cannot be broken when it comes to your children.

Sure, it's tough to deal with not being there in your kids's life every day. When you are around, you have to be careful not to cause too much confusion or any misunderstanding between you and your children.

You have to keep letting them know that you love them. You want them to be with you any time they're willing. They're always welcome. At the same time, you don't want to press yourself on them.

To me, it's like a chess game. One person has to move before the other one. And when that one person—your child—moves, you take the same step.

You walk with your child. Talk with your child. You be a responsible parent.

You have to take your arguments with the mother and put them aside. Children need two parents to feed and clothe them. So any arguments between you two are *not* important to them.

So I've got Dorian on my mind and my little boy on my mind. And one day I'm coming home from work and I find Kelly in bed with her ex-boyfriend—with my son there.

I lost my mind. I broke up stuff. The police came and at first arrested me for disorderly conduct. Lisa used that as an excuse to say I couldn't see Dorian, but I'd better keep sending a monthly support check. If I didn't, she'd take me to court.

I decided Kelly wasn't any better than Lisa. I moved out.

When I was twenty, my grandfather died. He was a deep down man, a *backbone* man. Whatever he did with work, first he made sure everybody at his home was all right. I decided I wanted to be that way, too.

I made a commitment to Lucy. We had a baby, a daughter, Tracy Leigh.

My favorite thing is to get all my kids together. The

other day, my two oldest started climbing on me, play wrestling. I played until my back got stiff. I tell them they're sisters and brothers, not half. Saying they're half only confuses them.

As your kids grow up, you've got to confront them. If you want them to have sense, talk to them like adults. My one-year-old, Tracy, can sit in front of the TV and remember a song off a commercial. That tells me she's ready to hear some about life and reality.

Lucy found a young fathers' program for me. I was ready to go. I opened up as soon as I started.

I only wondered why there aren't more programs. The ladies have their educational classes, their parenting classes. What young fathers have are people telling us, "You're not going to make it." That makes the young fathers I know fight even more to do better.

We all need help to make ourselves good role models for our kids. I've learned that a man can help make a baby. And a woman can have a baby. But a man and a woman can take care of children equally well.

"I'm beating the odds."

(CONTINUED FROM PART II, PREGNANT)

YVELINE, 21 YEARS OLD

You go through so much pain raising a child that the pain you went through giving birth can't compare.

 I was twelve when I had my daughter. I named her Katherine. At first, I didn't want to see her. I was going to give her up for adoption. Then I told the social worker, "I need more time."

 They made arrangements for me and Katherine to go into foster care. The problem was they couldn't find anyone who would take us together. She went one place; I went another.

 It was hard. Where I went there were other foster kids, an adopted one, and even grandchildren all in this one home. My first month I didn't talk to anyone. I turned the TV on to the soap operas, lay around, and ate.

 The second month I started talking, especially to Jay-Jay, a foster child who was now grown up. He told me, "People are going to put papers in front of you to sign away your child. Take time to think or you'll regret it."

 The social worker kept coming by. Sometimes I didn't even know what she was talking about. I was in another world. She wanted me to go into therapy. I said, "School will be my therapy."

 In March, I went back to seventh grade. There were only a couple of people that knew I was a mother. That was okay. I always thought everybody had a secret life. This was mine. Who knows what secrets others had.

One Saturday my foster nephew said there was a man at the door. It was my father. I hadn't spoken to him since I had my daughter. I was scared and happy and confused to see him. Once I told him what was going on, he said, "Of course, I don't hate you."

That same day, I called the social worker and told her, "Throw the adoption papers away. I'm keeping my daughter." I still cry with happiness when I think about that decision.

The social worker started telling me about shelters they had for teenage mothers and their children. The problem was I was thirteen, and back then you had to be fourteen to get in. Plus they had to have room.

When Katherine was almost a year old, I began to visit her every weekend. I had no idea how to be a mother. I hadn't seen her the whole time. All I had was her picture to carry in my wallet.

The day before my fourteenth birthday, Katherine and I were reunited. We moved into the New York Foundling Mother and Child Program, in the Bronx. It was like a house where there were mothers, their children, and a housemother.

The others had been with their children since giving birth. I didn't even know what to say to Katherine. And she was really quiet. I didn't blame her. She was two. She went from her foster home straight to me. I felt so dumb. Finally, I said, "Oh, well, I have to start being a mother."

I also decided I had to take advantage of everything that was available to teenage mothers. I wanted to make life better for me and my daughter. Then, once I got out on my own, I could keep on helping myself and show other people how to do it, too. My plan was to figure out how the *system* worked.

Here's what I discovered.

You can learn from other people. To do that you have

to build a network. This network is made up of other teenage parents. You want to know what they've found out. What help are they getting? What's WIC? Do they go to parenting classes? Do they have free medical care? Do they know where to buy discount kids' clothes? Whatever. And the next question is, where did they go to get that help?

Then you decide what you need, and go do the same.

You also want to build relationships with some trusted adults—social workers, a therapist, somebody like that. Why? Because they know things. If you show them you mean business, they'll help. But you can't just say, "Please, help me," and sit back and wait. You have to be optimistic and figure out what you want.

Maybe these adults don't have all the information you want right away, but they know how to get it. And if they don't know, they can find out.

For example, one time I found out that the school I was going to had a program where you work one week and go to school one week. I wanted to know how to get into that program. And if I did get in, could I save everything I earned? I wanted that money to go towards an apartment, and I wanted to find a cheap apartment as soon as possible.

See, I had this image of where I wanted to be in three years. I needed to find out, *How do I get there?* What does the city have to offer to HELP me get there? What was available to me before I turned eighteen? What was available after that?

Cassandra, a social worker, helped me a lot. I was lucky. Sometimes, though, the first person you ask won't pay much attention. Well, go to a second person or a third.

You have to do your own footwork, too. Double-check what they tell you. Sure, you get tired and frustrated. But there's always someone who'll help you. By getting help, you end up helping your child. That's what this is about: being a good parent.

You have to make your children your priority. You

BILLIONS AND BILLIONS

Last year the federal government spent more than $21.5 billion on welfare programs for families started by teenagers. State governments spent additional amounts.[10] To lower these costs, states have enacted or may enact these types of changes: reduce the amount of the monthly AFDC welfare check; replace welfare with jobs that pay below minimum wage; don't pay teen mothers extra money for each additional child; give a bonus to those who marry.[11]

have to be willing to sacrifice for them without being all droopy.

I'm not going to lie to you. I was not a totally boring teenager. I still went out. I still had sex. But, at the same time, I graduated from high school with flying colors. After four years at the Foundling, I moved into my own apartment in public housing—*finally*.

Katherine was six and I just turned eighteen. I knew I was starting college that fall. It would be hard. So that summer I was wild. Mind you, I still took care of business. My rule was, unless I was confident my daughter was fine, I wouldn't party.

I worked full time Monday through Friday 8:30 A.M. to 4:30 P.M. But every Friday night, Saturday night, and Sunday night that summer *I went out*. I went to clubs. I loved reggae music. I liked to talk to guys with nice cars. Come Monday, I was a zombie.

And then it was September. I became a college student.

I'm twenty-one now and a senior at Hunter College in New York City. I'm in a scholarship program, MARC, Minority Access to Research Careers. I have two part-time jobs, one at Citibank Tax Shelter and the other at Payne-Whitney Psychiatric Center. I plan to go to graduate school and, maybe, do research about AIDS among teenagers.

Katherine and I have a great relationship—more like sisters. I tell her, "Sure, we have a wonderful life together. But motherhood is harder than it seems." Where we live, we see mothers on drugs using their babies to beg for money. Katherine and I talk about things like that, too.

I remind her, I've never gotten pregnant a second time. There is no man, no love strong enough to make me have another child as a teenager.

I even tell her there are moments when I wonder what my life would have been like if I hadn't had her. "It's not like I regret having you," I say. "It's just that I *never* was a teenager. It must be fun."

But my Katherine *is* my life. I love watching her grow up.

I felt such satisfaction when she took her first step. I was so proud when she brought home her first 100 from school.

I thought, "Hey, I'm doing this right. I'm beating the odds against teen mothers." I'm putting a lot into being a good parent, but what I'm getting back is even greater. It keeps me moving. It's such a challenge.

I'm mushy with my daughter. I hug her a lot. I love to tell her I love her. And I just feel all her love in return. There's nothing else in the world quite like it, the love between a mother and child.

PART VII

Your Story

Name:
Age:

"WHAT STORY DO YOU WANT TO BE YOURS?"

On these pages you read other teenagers' stories. Before I closed this book on their lives, I gave some of them one more call. "How are you doing?" I asked.

Sarah [Part I: Sex], whose boyfriend was trying to trick her into having a baby, *did* become pregnant. Her first choice was to continue the pregnancy and have her parents raise the child. "Forget it," they told her.

Her boyfriend said he'd take over. Sarah decided that wasn't the best solution either. Next she considered adoption. Her mother pointed out that it wasn't black babies like hers, but healthy, white babies who were in demand.

Sarah saw abortion as the best answer. Her boyfriend promised to go with her. When Sarah and her mother stopped by to pick him up, no one came to the door. Later, he explained he'd run out to buy some milk.

Sarah and her boyfriend are still dating.

Remember Marisol [Part II: Pregnant]? Her birth control failed. She finished school the same night she went into labor. Today she's the "determined" mother of a baby boy.

"I have too much pride to sit home and live off hand-outs," she told me. "Anyway, I always wanted to go to college. Now I want to succeed for my son's sake, too."

This honor roll student plans to go to a community college first, then to a university to study international finance. A counselor is helping her get a scholarship. Marisol is sorry her boyfriend, Nicholas, had to quit school. They needed the money.

Courtney [Part II], the one living with Texas relatives, has "an adorable baby girl" and a new boyfriend, Josh. "I love the shit out of Josh," she said. "He's nineteen and has a two-year-old son in Arkansas. He doesn't see him much, but he sends money for toys and clothes."

She is taking her life in segments, not thinking about the future. "For now, I'll stay with my aunt and uncle, and take classes for teen mothers."

Kara [Part II], who very much wanted a baby, offered these highlights: Her boyfriend is no longer in the picture. The baby is due next week. After the birth, she'll go live with her sister. They reconnected after not having talked for the past two years.

Becky Bell's mother, Karen [Part III: Abortion], gave me this update: "One day my husband, Bill, was sitting in his office, staring at Becky's picture. I was in bed, crying. Our son said, Here's my sister lying in the grave. Mom, you've given up. Dad has given up. What do you think I feel like? Why don't you do something? Tell people what's happened to us.

"That's when we decided to go public. We talk to school groups, as well as state legislators who want to pass abortion parental consent and notification laws. We hope it helps those who hear us. It helps and hurts us.

"Right-to-lifers come up and say, 'We're sorry about the loss of your grandchild.' At first I didn't understand what they meant. I thought they were talking about Becky. But I was wrong. They don't acknowledge her.

"Now I say to them, 'You can be sorry about the loss of the fetus. We love and miss our little girl who was a living, beautiful seventeen-year-old.'"

Stephanie [Part IV: Foster Care] had placed her daughter, Rusty, in foster care. Three months later, the family said Rusty was too much to handle. She had to go to another.

Stephanie told them, "No way." Instead, Rusty went

to her cousins. "Last week I signed the papers so they can adopt her," Stephanie said. "I decided my life wasn't good enough for her to come back to me. Now I feel relieved because I know she's with a sweet, loving couple.

"At the same time, I feel sad. The love Rusty gave made me feel important. But I want her to make as much of herself as she can. I don't want her to go through all the crap I did. I'm optimistic."

Judy [Part IV], whose daughter's arm was broken, wasn't home when I called, but I talked to her sister. "Judy won't admit it," she said, "but for sure that was child abuse.

"They told her before she could get her baby back, she had to do a bunch of things like take parenting classes. Well, Judy didn't do them.

"That meant they took the baby away from her for good. Shannon's been adopted. Now here's the rumor. Judy has this new boyfriend, and I'm sure she's expecting."

Kristi [Part V: Adoption], whose boyfriend wasn't much help, had this to say: "Looking back, the only thing I regret is disappointing my parents. I think I handled the pregnancy and adoption well. I felt lucky. I gave two people who couldn't have kids the most precious thing in the world—a child.

"Now I've gotten to the point that if someone happens to find out about it, it's okay. It's part of my life. They'll have to deal with it.

"Then there's Kevin. I loved him. I wanted things to be back the way they were. But that didn't happen. About six months after the baby's birth, I started to date.

"I'm not very trusting anymore with guys. I don't want a relationship right now. But I did learn that if a relationship ends, it's not the end of your life."

Susan [Part VI: Parents] and her boyfriend, Peter, were always together. Now they're engaged. The big news, though, is that he's joined the army. When he couldn't find work in Texas, he saw that as his only option.

Susan and the baby, Misty, are going to join him for the summer in Georgia where he's stationed. Then she'll come back home and live with her parents while she finishes school.

When I asked her how her parents felt about all this, she said, "They don't care that we're not married. They know we will be when it matters."

Nicolette [Part VI] is still in her paternity battle with James. The results from the blood tests to determine if he's the father aren't back yet. She has another year before she graduates.

As for romance, she has a new boyfriend. Nicolette said, "After I had Pamela, I wanted to go out. My girlfriend fixed me up with this guy, Adam. When I told him I had a baby, I thought he'd turn away. He didn't. He cares for the baby. She smiles when she sees him. He changes and feeds her.

"I love Adam. I don't think I ever loved James. Adam says he's going to ask me to marry him. I think I'll tell him, yes."

In the first chapter, I wrote, "This is a book more of stories than statistics." But now in the last chapter, let's also look at some numbers and the stories they tell:

If you don't wait until your twenties to have children, the odds are against you and your baby. You both may suffer.

- The babies of teenage mothers are more likely to be premature or not weigh very much at birth.[1] And when that happens, the chances are greater that they will die during their first year, have birth injuries, serious childhood illness, and nerve defects—including mental retardation.[2]
- Soon you discover that caring for your children often becomes your full-time job. It IS hard to be both a good parent and continue your education. In fact,

eight out of ten who have babies at seventeen or younger drop out of high school.[3] Only one in fifty graduates from college.[4]

• A college degree is no guarantee that you'll be a perfect parent or that you'll be able to support your child. But with limited education, not much job experience, a small child or two to look after, and usually no husband to help, statistics show that most teenage mothers are forced to turn to public assistance to keep the family together.

• Families headed by teen mothers are seven times more likely than others to be poor. The younger the mother when she gives birth, the lower her family income.[5] And you know what happens when money's tight. You can't do for your kids the way you want to.

• Now here's one last statistic: Those who give birth at fifteen or sixteen are likely to have at least one other child before they turn twenty.[6]

None of this means that you can't or you won't be the best parent around. It does mean, though, you have an uphill battle to prove that in your case, those numbers don't tell the whole story.

You are special and unique. You can decide today you want to write your success story. To start with, you could say, "I'll do what I have to do to avoid a surprise pregnancy."

But if that doesn't happen—and you rule out abortion or adoption—you can still decide to beat the odds against teen mothers. The choice is yours.

Teen men have choices, too. You can get a partner pregnant and leave. Or you can say, "That baby's part of me, too. I'm mature enough to be responsible for another life."

What story do you want to be yours?

GLOSSARY

ADC/AFDC: Aid for Families with Dependent Children, a federal program that provides monthly income to pay for the expenses of children of people who have an income below certain poverty guidelines

amniotic fluid: the liquid or "water" in which the fetus floats throughout the pregnancy

Caesarian section/C-section: delivery of a child by means of surgical incisions (cuts) through abdominal wall and uterus

ectopic pregnancy/tubal pregnancy: ectopic means "out of place"; a pregnancy where the fertilized ovum (egg) implants somewhere outside the uterus in the abdominal cavity. When the ovum implants in a fallopian tube, it is called a tubal pregnancy.

epidural: local anesthetic given when the female is in labor prior to childbirth

episiotomy: small, surgical incision made in the (perineal) tissue to enlarge the opening of the vagina for ease in delivery

fallopian tubes: tubes that carry the ripened ovum (egg) from the female's ovaries to her uterus; the tubes go from near each ovary to the uterus

maternity: related to mothering, and being a mother

ovaries: female sex glands which produce the ripened ovum ready to be fertilized by male sperm

paternity: related to fathering, and being a father

prenatal care: regular medical care prior to the birth

pro-choice: supports the idea that women have a right to an abortion if they choose to have one

pro-life: anti-abortion; supports the idea that women have no right to an abortion

trimester: pregnancy is divided into three parts: the first trimester is about weeks 1 to 13; the second is about weeks 14 to 25; the third is about weeks 26 to 38

umbilical cord: a ropelike cord, filled with blood vessels, that connects the fetus to the placenta

SOURCE NOTES

PART I: SEX

1. Michael J. Clark, "Complaints Prompt Howard Co. Schools to Evaluate 2 Books," *The Baltimore Sun*, 23 October 1990, Maryland section.
2. Nadine Joseph, Pamela G. Kripke, Binnie Fisher, and Regina Elam, "The New Rules for Courtship," *Newsweek Special Issue*, Summer/Fall 1990, p. 27. Figures reflect only teens in metropolitan areas. Source—females: National Survey of Family Growth; males: Urban Institute.
3. Philip J. Hilts, "Birth Control Safer than Unprotected Sex," *New York Times*, 4 April 1991, Science section. Report by Alan Guttmacher Institute to show a statistical picture of contraception in America.
4. Barbara Kantrowitz, "The Dangers of Doing It," *Newsweek Special Issue*, Summer/Fall 1990, p. 56–57.
5. Laurie Garrett, "Issue: Fighting AIDS. Why Teens Are At Risk," *New York Newsday*, 6 August 1991, Student Briefing Page.
6. Mireya Navarro, "Women With AIDS Virus: Hard Choices on Motherhood," *New York Times*, 23 July 1991, Metropolitan section.
7. Alan Guttmacher Institute, "Teenage Pregnancy: The Problem that Hasn't Gone Away," New York, 1981.

PART II: PREGNANT

1. Telephone inquiry, 31 July 1991, Alan Guttmacher Institute, 1987 most recent year available. (Exact number 1,014,620.)

2. AP wire service, "Panel Urges Consolidation of Prenatal Care," *New York Times*, 24 April 1991, National section. Report by National Commission to Prevent Infant Mortality. Alan Guttmacher Institute, "Teenage Pregnancy: The Problem that Hasn't Gone Away," New York, 1981.

3. Margaret Carlson, "Abortion's Hardest Cases," *Time*, 9 July 1990, p. 24.

4. Jane E. Brody, "Allergies in Infants Are Linked to Mothers' Diets," *New York Times*, 30 August 1990, Health section.

5. Ibid.

6. Robert Coles, "Girl Scouts Survey on the Beliefs and Moral Values of America's Children," New York: GSUSA, Fall 1989, p. 51–52.

7. Mary Cronin, Melissa Ludtke, and James Willwerth, "Innocent Victims," *Time*, 13 May 1991, p. 57.

8. Coles, op. cit., p. 51.

PART III: ABORTION

1. Natalie Angier, "Study Says Anger Troubles Women Denied Abortions," *New York Times*, 29 May 1991, Health section. Study by Paul K.B. Dagg, M.D., Mount Sinai Hospital, Toronto, Canada.

2. Margaret Carlson, "Abortion's Hardest Cases," *Time*, 9 July 1990, p. 24.

3. Ann Thompson Cook, "Fact Sheet—Safety of Abortion," National Abortion Federation.

4. Kim Painter, "'87 Abortion Rate Shows Decline From '80," *USA Today*, 25 April 1991, p. 1. Report by Alan Guttmacher Institute.

5. Heather Pearson and her mother became involved

in a lawsuit where they tried to have the Minnesota parental notification law thrown out. The case ended up before the United States Supreme Court. The law was upheld. It still stands.

6. Tamar Lewin, "Abortions Harder to Get in Rural Areas of Nation," *New York Times*, 28 June 1990. Survey by Alan Guttmacher Institute, figures from 1988.

PART IV: FOSTER CARE

1. Neil A. Lewis, "US Judge Rules District of Columbia Is Abusing Rights of Foster Children," *New York Times*, 19 April 1991, National section.

2. AP wire service, "Study Finds Severe Effects From Childhood Abuse," *New York Times*, 18 February 1991, National section. Studies by Cathy Spatz Widom, State University of New York at Albany; Byron Egeland, University of Minnesota.

3. J.C. Barden, "Foster Care System Reeling, Despite Law Meant to Help," *New York Times*, 21 September 1990, National section.

PART V: ADOPTION

1. Dirk Johnson, "Case of Abandoned Boy Brings Look at Adoption," *New York Times*, 22 April 1990, National section. Figures from David S. Liederman, executive director, Child Welfare League of America.

2. Alan Guttmacher Institute, Facts in Brief, "Teenage Sexual and Reproductive Behavior in the United States," 1987 most recent year available.

3. Elizabeth Kolbert, "Fathers' Rights on Adoption Are Expected," *New York Times*, 11 July 1990.

4. Katherine Bishop, "A Yearning for Psychic Wholeness—For the Adopted, the Issue of Roots Grows Stronger," *New York Times*, 7 October 1990, Week in Review section. Nationwide, there are an estimated 5 million

adoptees. According to William L. Pierce, president, National Committee for Adoption, no more than one in five adoptees seek their birth parents.

5. Johnson, op. cit.

PART VI: PARENTS

1. Felicity Barringer, "After Long Decline, Teen Births Are Up," *New York Times*, 17 August 1990, National section. Report from the National Center for Health Statistics.

2. Telephone inquiry, 10 May 1991, National Center for Health Statistics, 1988 most recent year available.

3. Telephone inquiry, 10 May 1991, Alan Guttmacher Institute, 1987 most recent year available.

4. J. Dustin Nichols, "A Garden Regained," *New York Times Magazine*, 12 May 1991, Letters, p. 12.

5. Tamar Lewin, "Father's Vanishing Act Called Common Drama," *New York Times*, 4 June 1990, National section. Study by Frank Furstenberg and Kathleen Mullan Harris, University of Pennsylvania.

6. Nancy Gibbs, "Shameful Bequests to the Next Generation," *Time*, 8 October 1990, p. 43.

7. AP wire service, "Cow Antibodies Are Linked to Colic in Babies," *New York Times*, 30 March 1991.

8. Elisabeth Rosenthal, "Measles Resurges, and With Deadlier Effects," *New York Times*, 24 April 1991, National section. Data from National Centers for Disease Control.

9. Daniel Goleman, "Parent Is Seen as Key to Happiness," *New York Times*, 18 April 1991. Study by Dr. Carol Franz, psychologist, Boston University.

10. AP wire service, "US Spent $21.5 Billion in 1989 to Support Families of Teen-Agers," *New York Times*, 24 September 1990, National section. Report by the Center for Population Options.

11. Jason DeParle, "As Funds for Welfare Shrink, Ideas Flourish," *New York Times*, 12 May 1991, Week in Review section.

PART VII: YOUR STORY

1. AP wire service, "Panel Urges Consolidation of Prenatal Care," *New York Times*, 24 April 1991, National section.

2. "Substantially Higher Morbidity and Mortality Rates Found Among Infants Born to Adolescent Mothers," Family Planning Perspective, Vol. 16, 1984. The Alan Guttmacher Institute.

3. Margaret Carlson, "Abortion's Hardest Cases," *Time*, 9 July 1990, p. 25.

4. Telephone inquiry, 10 May 1991, Alan Guttmacher Institute.

5. Ibid.

6. Alan Guttmacher Institute, "Teenage Pregnancy: The Problem that Hasn't Gone Away," New York, 1981.

FOR FURTHER READING

Bell, Ruth. *Changing Bodies, Changing Lives: A Book for Teens on Sex and Relationships*, revised edition. New York: Vintage Books, 1988. (Young Adult)

Bettelheim, Bruno. *A Good Enough Parent: A Book on Childrearing*. New York: Alfred Knopf, 1987. (Adult)

Brazelton, T. Berry. *Working and Caring*. Reading, Mass.: Addison-Wesley Pub. Co., 1985. (A)

Brown, Fern G. *Teen Guide To Childbirth*. New York: Franklin Watts, 1988. (YA)

Calderone, Mary S., and Eric W. Johnson. *The Family Book About Sexuality*, revised edition. New York: Harper and Row, 1989. (YA & A)

Dash, Leon. *When Children Want Children: The Urban Crisis of Teenage Childbearing*. New York: William Morrow, 1989. (A)

Dorris, Michael. *The Broken Cord: A Family's Ongoing Struggle with Fetal Alcohol Syndrome*. New York: Harper & Row, 1989. (A)

DuPrau, Jeanne. *Adoption: The Facts, Feelings, and Issues of a Double Heritage*. Englewood Cliffs, N.J.: Julian Messner, 1990. (YA)

Emmens, Carol A. *The Abortion Controversy*. New York: Julian Messner, 1987. (YA)

Firestone, Robert. *Compassionate Child-Rearing: An In-Depth Approach to Optimal Parenting*. New York: Insight Books, 1990. (A)

Guernsey, JoAnn Bren. *Teen Pregnancy*. New York: Clarion Books, 1989. (YA)

Harding, Edith, and Philip Riley. *The Bilingual Family: A Handbook for Parents*. New York. Cambridge University Press, 1986. (A)

Herzfeld, Judith. *Sense and Sensibility in Childbirth*. New York: W.W. Norton, 1985. (A)

Jakobson, Cathryn. *Think About: Teenage Pregnancy*. New York: Walker, 1988. (YA)

Levant Ronald F., and John Kelly. *Between Father and Son: How To Become the Kind of Father You Want To Be*. New York: Viking, 1989. (A)

Lindsay, Jeanne Warren. *Open Adoption: A Caring Option*. Buena Park, Calif.: Morning Glory Press, 1987. (YA)

Nourse, Alan E. *Teen Guide to Safe Sex*. New York: Franklin Watts, 1988. (YA)

Orr, Lisa, editor. *Sexual Values*. San Diego, Calif.: Greenhaven, 1989. (YA)

Ross, Anne G. *Teenage Mothers, Teenage Fathers*. Toronto, Canada, and Edison, N.J.: Everest House, 1982. (YA)

Silverstein, Herma. *Teenage and Pregnant: What You Can Do*. Englewood Cliffs, N.J.: Julian Messner, 1988. (YA)

Spock, Benjamin. *Baby and Childcare*, revised edition, New York: Dutton, 1985. (A)

Terkel, Susan Neiburg. *Abortion: Facing the Issues*, New York: Franklin Watts, 1988. (YA)

Vecchiolla, Francine, and Penelope L. Maza. *Pregnant and Parenting Adolescents*. Washington, D.C.: Children's Welfare League, 1989. (A)

Worth, Cecilia. *The Birth of a Father: New Fathers Talk About Pregnancy, Childbirth, and the First Three Months*. New York: McGraw-Hill, 1988. (A)

Zollar, Ann Creighton. *Adolescent Pregnancy and Parenthood: An Annotated Guide*. New York: Garland, 1990. (A)

INDEX

ABOUT THE AUTHOR

Janet Bode specializes in writing nonfiction books for teenagers. Across the country, she asks students about the critical issues they face today. Then, to find guidance for the problems the students raise, she interviews professionals and experts on these specific topics. The result is a series of hard-hitting, award-winning books that combine revealing, teen-life stories with perceptive analysis and workable solutions. The titles of these Watts publications include *Different Worlds: Interracial and Cross-Cultural Dating; New Kids on the Block: Oral Histories of Immigrant Teens; The Voices of Rape; Truce: Ending the Sibling War;* and *Beating the Odds: Stories of Unexpected Achievers.* In addition, Bode has written two books for the adult market and numerous articles for such national periodicals as *Glamour, Cosmopolitan, Mademoiselle, Savvy,* and *Redbook.*

A lifelong traveler, Ms. Bode has lived and worked in the United States, Europe, and Mexico. She now resides in New York City, where she is a member of the Authors Guild and PEN.